OMT Review

Second Edition

Copyright © 1998, 1999 by Robert G. Savarese, D.O.

2nd printing: March 2000

To purchase a copy of OMT Review for $25.95, or comments, questions, and suggestions, please send e-mail to the author at omtreview@hotmail.com

Reprints of chapters may be purchased from Robert Savarese at omtreview@hotmail.com

ISBN: 0-9670090-0-6

Printed in the United States of America

Notice: the authors of this volume have taken care to make certain that the information contained herein is correct and compatible with the standards generally accepted at the time of the publication. As new information becomes available, changes in treatment modalities invariably follow; therefore when choosing a particular treatment, the reader should consider not only the information provided in this manual but also any recently published medical literature on the subject. The nature of this text is to be a comprehensive review, but due to the extraordinary amount of material it is beyond the scope of this text to include all aspects of Osteopathic Medicine. It is advised that the reader familiarizes himself with the information contained in one of the excellent osteopathic texts that form the cornerstone of osteopathic medical education. Lastly, the authors and distributors disclaims any liability, loss, injury, or damage incurred as a consequence, directly or indirectly, of the use and application of any of the contents of this volume.

OMT Review

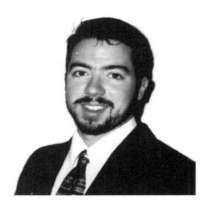

Author and Editor-in Chief

Robert G. Savarese, D.O.

Osteopathic Fellow
Graduate of Nova Southeastern University
Kessler Institute for Rehabilitation
Dept. of Physical Medicine and Rehabilitation
West Orange, NJ

Medical illustration by
Robert G. Savarese, D.O.

Contributing Authors

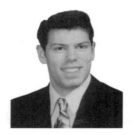

Glenn S. Fuoco, D.O.

Chapter 16 "Special Tests"
Graduate of Philadelphia College of Osteopathic Medicine
Baylor College of Medicine
Department of Physical Medicine and Rehabilitation
Houston, Texas

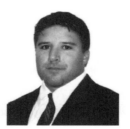

Daniel G. Berson, D.O.

Chapter 13 "Muscle Energy"
Osteopathic Fellow
Graduate of Nova Southeastern University
University of Florida
Dept. of Anesthesiology
Ft. Lauderdale, FL

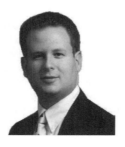

Marc Kaprow

Co-author of COMLEX Style Examination
Osteopathic Fellow
Nova Southeastern University
College of Osteopathic Medicine
Ft. Lauderdale, FL

Who can use this book?

1. Anyone interested in Osteopathic (Manual) Medicine

   Practicing clinicians (M.D. or D.O.), occupational or physical therapists can utilize the information and techniques in this book to further their knowledge in osteopathic medicine.

2. 1st and 2nd year medical students

   For those students using this text as a quick reference to study from during the first two years of medical school, keep in mind that diagnosis and treatment vary from practitioner to practitioner and by school to school. Although this book reflects the "Foundations" book, certain types of techniques may be taught differently at your school. It is therefore important to use class notes as well as this text while studying for examinations throughout the first two years.

3. Studying for COMLEX Step 1, 2 and 3

   This book is currently the only comprehensive review book for OMT. This book is designed to eliminate the need of sifting through old OMT notes when studying for the COMLEX boards. For those students comfortable with their knowledge of OMT, it may prove beneficial to start with the comprehensive examination. Hone in on weak areas, then study those chapters in the book. Also, focus on the autonomic reflexes in chapter 9, "Facilitation". Many board questions will stem from this area.

4. Last minute cramming

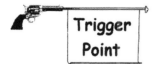 The information contained in the gray shaded box following this symbol is important. Trigger Points are main concepts. For those individuals cramming for exams, Trigger Points help the reader to pull out key information quickly.

NOTE: The information contained in the gray shaded box following this symbol does not have any relation to Travell's triggerpoint (see chapter 10). The Trigger Point symbol in this text is merely a method of highlighting important information

Dedication

To Melissa,
For her genuine support and understanding,
without which this book never could have been completed.

To my parents,
Who taught me about hard work and perseverance

Acknowledgments

―――――――――――――――――――――

Although this book was a task undertaken by one person, in reality it is a compilation of the knowledge and ideas from colleagues, experts, and friends. I wish to extend special thanks to the following people:

Glenn S. Fuoco, D.O., Daniel G. Berson, D.O., and Marc Kaprow, who demonstrated enthusiasm and determination toward their contribution to this book. Thank you very much for the long hours spent putting together your chapters.

Mark Sandhouse, D.O., whose extraordinary academic knowledge, and particular attention to detail, ensured the future readers of this book correct information in a concise format.

Ronald B. Tolchin, D.O., and Jan Garrison, M.D., who both have played an integral role in my development as a medical student

John Capobianco, D.O. who gave me insight about how osteopathic medicine is presented to students at other schools. John thank you very much, your knowledge has helped <u>OMT Review</u> become a textbook accepted throughout the nation.

The entire OMM faculty and fellows at NSU, whose wisdom, insight and guidance allowed me to write a book that is a comprehensive review of important osteopathic principles.

Melissa Krueger, for her love and support and the many hours spent revising the final manuscripts. I would also like to thank her for the time spent modeling for the photographs.

Nishith Jobanputra, D.O., M.P.H., who was kind enough to help with proofreading the manuscript.

Nancy Beckhorn whose particular attention to detail helped me fine tune the text.

Tom Fotopoulos who helped research important facts.

Christine Chapman who dedicated many hours revising the COMLEX style examination.

To all clinical and academic professors, who have imparted their knowledge upon myself and other medical students, in order to improve health care and further osteopathic medical education. Thank you.

Robert G. Savarese, D.O.

Preface

During the first two years of my medical training, the need for a comprehensive OMT review book became increasingly apparent. Every year, thousands of osteopathic medical students are left sifting through 2 years of OMT notes, or reading various texts, in order to study for the OMT section of the boards.

This book was written to reflect the current understanding and knowledge of osteopathic medicine as written in the <u>Foundations</u> <u>for</u> <u>Osteopathic</u> <u>Medicine</u> and the many other texts which form the cornerstone of osteopathic medical education. The <u>Foundations</u> <u>for</u> <u>Osteopathic</u> <u>Medicine</u>, published in 1997, established itself as standardized text for the education of osteopathic medical students. The "Foundations" text serve a primary source-book from which questions are written for the COMLEX examinations.

<u>OMT</u> <u>Review</u> is in not intended to substitute for any of the excellent osteopathic reference texts. It is intended to be used as quick reference as well as a board review. A combination of basic osteopathic principles along with important clinical points makes this book useful for osteopathic medical students as well as anyone interested in osteopathic medicine. It is hoped that the concise style, tables, and illustrations help summarize and enhance the readers' recollection of principle points. The comprehensive examination at the end of the book will help students gauge their progress, and focus their efforts with maximum efficiency.

It is my sincere wish that this book will serve as a source through which its readers can rapidly grasp the fundamental principles of osteopathic medicine.

Robert G. Savarese, D.O.

Table of Contents

Chapter 1
The Basics

I. Somatic dysfunction

A. Definition - *Somatic dysfunction is an impairment or altered function of related components of the somatic (body framework) system: skeletal, arthroidial, and myofascial structures and related vascular, lymphatic and neural elements.* [1 p.1138]

In simpler terms: Somatic dysfunction is a restriction that can occur in bones joints, muscle, fascia. Blood supply, lymph flow and nervous function may be altered in somatic dysfunction.

B. Diagnostic criteria

Somatic dysfunction is a **R**estriction,
but can also present itself as:

Tenderness

Asymmetry

Tissue texture changes

An easy way to remember this is to use the mnemonic: **TART.**

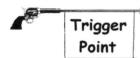

Trigger Point	**Know what TART stands for.**

1. Tenderness - may be produced during palpation of tissues where it should not occur if there was no somatic dysfunction.

2. Asymmetry - bones, muscles, or joints may feel asymmetric to the corresponding structures.

3. Restriction (see fig 1.1a and 1.1b) - a joint in somatic dysfunction will have restricted motion. Under normal physiologic conditions a joint has two barriers:
   a. **Physiologic barrier** - a point at which a patient can actively move any given joint. For example, a person may actively rotate his head 80° to either side.
   b. **Anatomic barrier** - a point at which a physician can passively move any given joint. For example, a physician may passively rotate the same patient's head 90° to either side.
   NOTE: any movement beyond the anatomical barrier will cause ligament, tendon, or skeletal injury.
   c. In somatic dysfunction, a joint will have a **restrictive (or pathologic) barrier** (see fig 1.1b). A restrictive barrier lies before the physiologic barrier, and prevents full range of motion of that joint. For example, a patient may have a full range of motion for rotation of the neck to the right. However, the patient may only be able to turn his head to the left approximately 70°. Therefore, a restrictive barrier is met when turning the head to the left.

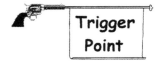

Trigger Point

Know the difference between physiologic, anatomic and restrictive barriers

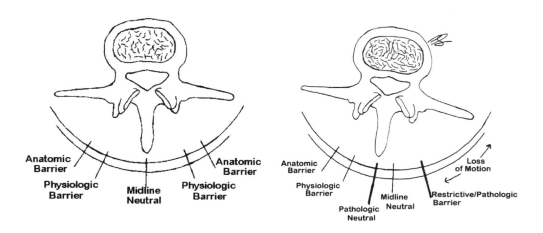

Fig 1.1a (left): In a vertebral segment without somatic dysfunction the vertebrae may rotate equally to either side. Fig 1.1b (right): If somatic dysfunction is present, the vertebral segment will not lie in the midline position, and the patient will not be able to rotate the vertebral segment past the restrictive (or pathologic) barrier.

4. Tissue texture changes - may present in many ways. The surrounding tissue may be edematous, tender, fibrosed, atrophied, rigid, or hypertonic.

C. **Differences between acute and chronic somatic dysfunction**

TART findings will be altered as an injury changes from acute to chronic. Table 1.1 describes findings in acute vs. chronic somatic dysfunction. [1 p.476, 2 p.9]

Table 1.1

Findings	Acute	Chronic
Tenderness	Severe, sharp	Dull, achy, burning
Asymmetry	Present.	Present with compensation in other areas of the body.
Restriction	Present, painful with movement	Present, decreased or no pain.
Tissue texture changes	Edematous, erythematous, boggy with increased moisture. Muscles hypertonicy	Decreased or no edema, no erythema, cool dry skin, with slight tension. Decreased muscle tone, flaccid, ropy, fibrotic

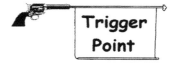

Trigger Point

Know the findings regarding acute and chronic somatic dysfunction.

II. Fryette's Principles

A. Principle I

In 1918 Harrison Fryette noted, with the use of radiographs, that there were certain rules to spinal motion. Fryette combined the principles of somatic dysfunction and these rules to establish what are now regarded as Fryette's principles. Fryette's principles act as guidelines for physicians to discriminate different types of dysfunctions, and to determine diagnoses.

Fryette first noticed that *if the spine is in the neutral position (no flexion or extension), and if sidebending is introduced, rotation would then occur to the opposite side.* For example, if a person were to sidebend to the left so that L2 can no longer sidebend on L3 (the facets are locked), then L2 will start to rotate to the right in order to facilitate further sidebending. Fryette then applied this rule to the principles of somatic dysfunction. He noticed if L2 is in the neutral position and restricted in left rotation, then L2 is rotated right and ***must*** be sidebent left. This became Fryette's principle I.

Summary of Principle I

◊   In the neutral position:
*sidebending precedes rotation,
sidebending and rotation occur to
opposite sides.*

◊   Fryette used this principle for
nomenclature of somatic dysfunction:
      e.g.: NS_LR_R or NSR_R = neutral,
      sidebent left, rotated right.

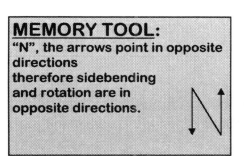

MEMORY TOOL:
"N", the arrows point in opposite directions
therefore sidebending and rotation are in opposite directions.

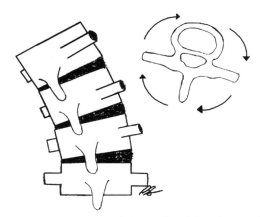

Fig 1.2:Fryette's principle I: Left sidebending without flexion or extension will cause right rotation of all vertebrae.

B. Principle II

Fryette then noticed that if the spine is in the non-neutral position (either flexed or extended), and rotation is introduced, sidebending would then occur to the same side. For example, if a person were to rotate to the left so that L2 can no longer rotate on L3 (the facets are locked), then L2 will start to sidebend to the left in order to facilitate further rotation. He applied this rule to somatic dysfunction, and noticed if L2 is either flexed or extended and restricted in left rotation, then L2 is rotated right and *must* be sidebent right. This became Fryette's principle II.

Summary of Principle II
◊   In a non-neutral (flexed or
      extended) position:
*rotation precedes sidebending,
sidebending and rotation occur to the
same side.*

◊   Fryette used this principle for
nomenclature of somatic dysfunction:
      e.g.: FR_RS_R or FRS_R = flexed,
      rotated and sidebent right.

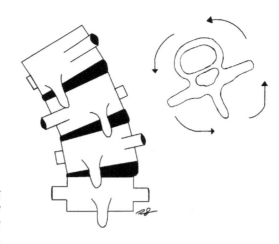

*Fig 1.3: Fryette's principle II: Left sidebending
with flexion or extension will cause one
vertebrae to rotate and sidebend to the same
side.*

MEMORY TOOL:
In "F"lexed or "E"xtended lesions the arrows point in the same direction therefore rotation and sidebending are the same direction.

Principle I is typical of group dysfunctions.
      For example: L2-L5 NS_RR_L or NSR_L.
Principle II is typical of a single vertebral dysfunction.
      For example: T5 FR_RS_R or FRS_R.

NOTE:
Fryette's principles I and II only apply to the thoracic and lumbar vertebrae!!
Not the cervical vertebrae!!

C. Principle III:
Initiating motion of any vertebral segment in any one plane of motion will influence the mobility of that segment in the other two planes of motion. [1 p.1138] For example, forward bending will decrease the ability to sidebend and rotate.

III. Naming and evaluating somatic dysfunction
A. Naming somatic dysfunctions
As mentioned above, somatic dysfunction is diagnosed by **TART** (tenderness, asymmetry, restriction, and tissue texture changes). When evaluating somatic dysfunction the physician will examine all of these components, especially restriction. Evaluation of restriction will allow the physician to diagnose and name the somatic dysfunction.

In the case of vertebral segments, motion will occur in flexion/extension, rotation and sidebending to either side. Therefore, restriction can occur in any of these three planes. When referring to segmental motion, or restriction, *it is traditional to refer to motion (or restriction) of the segment **above** in a functional vertebral unit (two vertebrae)*. For example, when describing the motion (or restriction) of L2, it is the motion (or restriction) of L2 on top of L3.

Somatic dysfunctions are always named for their freedom of motion.

Three examples:

1. If L2 is restricted in the motions of flexion, sidebending to the right and rotation to the right, then L2 is said to be extended, rotated and sidebent to the left on L3. This is denoted as L2 ER_LS_L or ERS_L.

2. If T5 is restricted in the motions of extension, sidebending to the left and rotating to the left then, T5 is said to be flexed, rotated and sidebent to the right on T6. This is denoted as T5 FR_RS_R or FRS_R.

3. If T1 is not restricted in flexion or extension, but is restricted in sidebending to the left and rotating to the right, then T1 is said to be neutral, sidebent right and rotated left. This is denoted as NSR_L or NS_RR_L.

B. <u>Evaluating somatic dysfunctions</u>

<u>Cervical spine</u>

See chapter 2 Cervical Spine section D "Motion testing".

<u>Thoracic and lumbar spine</u>

1. **Assess rotation by placing the thumbs over the transverse processes of each segment.**
   If the right thumb is more posterior than the left, then the segment is rotated right.

2. **Then check the rotation of the segment in flexion.**
   If the rotation gets better (i.e. the right thumb is no longer posterior), this suggests that the segment is flexed, sidebent and rotated right FR_RS_R.

3. **Then check the segment in extension.**
   If the rotation gets better in extension, this suggests that the segment is extended, sidebent and rotated right ER_RS_R.
   If the rotation remains the same in flexion and extension, then the segment is neutral sidebent left and rotated right NS_LR_R.

IV. <u>Facet orientation and spinal motion</u>

A. <u>Orientation of SUPERIOR facets</u>

Facet orientation will determine the motion of the vertebral segments. For example, if a pair of facets were to face backward and medial, then sagittal plane motion would be favored (flexion and extension). An easy mnemonic to remember the orientation of superior facets in the axial skeleton is shown in table 1.2

Table 1.2

Region	Facet Orientation	mnemonic
Cervical	backward, upward, medial	**BUM**
Thoracic	backward, upward, lateral	**BUL**
Lumbar	backward, medial	**BM**

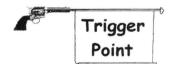

Trigger Point

Know the superior facets orientation.

B. Physiologic motion of the spine

The human spine can move in three planes or any combination thereof. Each plane corresponds with a particular axis and motion shown in table 1.3.

Table 1.3

motion	axis	plane
flx'n/ext'n	transverse	sagittal
rotation	vertical	transverse
sidebending	anterior - posterior	coronal

V.   Muscle contraction

A.   Isotonic contraction - Muscle contraction that results in the approximation of the muscle's origin and insertion without a change in its tension. In such a case the operator's force is less than the patient's force. [1 p.693, p.1129]

B.   Isometric contraction - Muscle contraction that results in the increase in tension without an approximation of origin and insertion.. In such a case the operator's force and the patient's force are equal. [1 p.693 p.1129]

C.   Isolytic contraction - Muscle contraction against resistance while forcing the muscle to lengthen. In such a case the operator's force is more than the patient's force. [1 p.693 p.1129]

D.   Concentric contraction - Muscle contraction that results in the approximation of the muscle's origin and insertion. [1 p.693 p.1129]

E.   Eccentric contraction - Lengthening of muscle during contraction due to an external force. [1 p.693 p.1129]

VI. Osteopathic Treatment

A. Direct vs. Indirect treatment

As mentioned earlier, all somatic dysfunctions will have a restrictive (pathologic) barrier. This restrictive barrier will inhibit movement in one direction thus causing asymmetry within the joint or tissue. The goal of osteopathic treatment is to eliminate this restrictive barrier, thus restoring symmetry.

Osteopathic practitioners use a variety of treatments to achieve this goal. All of these treatments fall into two categories, **direct treatment** and **indirect treatment**.

In a direct treatment, the practitioner "engages" the restrictive barrier. This means that the body tissues and/or joints are moved closer to the restrictive barrier. This can be done by direct palpation of the dysfunctional tissues or using a body part as a lever.

For example:
1.   If T3 was $FR_R S_R$, the practitioner would extend, rotate and sidebend T3 to the left.
2.   If the abdominal fascia moved more freely cephalad than caudad, the practitioner would hold the tissue caudad (toward the barrier) allowing the tissues to stretch.

In an indirect treatment the practitioner moves tissues and/or joints away from the restrictive barrier.

For example:
1.   If T3 was $FR_R S_R$, the practitioner would flex, sidebend and rotate T3 to the right.
2.   If the abdominal fascia moved more freely cephalad than caudad, the practitioner would hold the tissue cephalad (away from the barrier) allowing the tissues to relax.

B. Passive vs. Active Treatment

◊   *In an active treatment, the patient will assist in the treatment, usually in the form of isometric or isotonic contraction.*

◊   *In a passive treatment, the patient will relax and allow the practitioner to move the body tissues.*

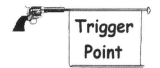

Trigger Point

Direct Treatment:	**Towards the barrier**
Indirect Treatment:	**Away from the barrier**
Active Treatment:	**Patient assists during treatment**
Passive Treatment:	**Patient relaxes during treatment**

Table 1.4

Treatment type	Direct or indirect	Active or passive
Myofascial Release	Both	Both
Counterstrain	Indirect	Passive
Facilitated Positional Release	Indirect	Passive
Muscle Energy	Direct (rarely indirect)	Active
High Velocity Low Amplitude	Direct	Passive

VII. Treatment Plan

A. Choice of Treatment

Precise answers to choice of technique do not exist; there are only general guidelines. [1 p.486]

1. Elderly patients and hospitalized patients typically respond better with indirect techniques or gentle direct techniques such as articulatory techniques.
2. The use of HVLA in a patient with advanced osteoporosis may lead to a pathologic fracture. [1 p.486]
3. Acute neck strain/sprains are often better treated with indirect techniques to prevent further strain.
4. Patients with advanced stages of cancer should not be treated with lymphatic techniques due to the increased risk of lymphogenous spread. [1 p.428]

B. Dose and Frequency

Absolute rules for dose and frequency do not exist. Typical guidelines are as follows: [1 p.486]

1. The sicker the patient the less the dose.
2. Allow time for the patient to respond to the treatment.
3. Chronic disease requires chronic treatment.
4. Pediatric patients can be treated more frequently; geriatric patients need a longer interval to respond to the treatment.
5. Acute cases should have a shorter interval between treatments; as they respond, the interval in increased.

C. Sequencing of Treatment

There are different opinions regarding what should be treated first. Guidelines on sequencing are not absolute. Each physician after gaining experience develops his or her own approach. The following is a sample sequence: [1 p.485-6]

1. For low back pain, and especially with psoas involvement, treat the lumbar spine first.
2. Treat the upper thoracic spine and ribs before treating the cervical spine.
3. Treat the thoracic spine before treating specific rib dysfunctions.
4. For very acute somatic dysfunctions, treat secondary or peripheral areas to allow access to the acute area.
5. Cranial treatment can produce relaxation and allow OMT to work in the other areas.
6. For extremity problems, treat the axial skeletal components first (spine, sacrum, ribs).

Chapter 2
Cervical Spine

I. Anatomy

A. Bones

The cervical spine consists of seven vertebral segments (see fig 2.1). C1 and C2 are considered atypical. C1 has no spinous process or vertebral body. C2 has a dens that projects superiorly from its body and articulates with C1. C2 - C6 have bifid spinous processes. The articular pillars (or lateral masses) are the portion of bone of the cervical vertebral segments that lie between the superior and inferior facets. The articular pillars are located posterior to the cervical transverse processes, and are used by osteopathic physicians to evaluate cervical vertebral motion. Foramen transversarium are foramina in the transverse process of C1-C6 that allow for the passage of the vertebral artery.

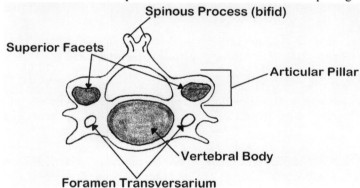

Spinous Process (bifid)

Superior Facets

Articular Pillar

Vertebral Body

Foramen Transversarium

Fig 2.1: A typical cervical vertebrae

B. Muscles

Scalenes (anterior, middle, posterior) - sidebend the neck to the same side with unilateral contraction, and flex the neck with bilateral contraction. The scalenes also aid in respiration. *The anterior and middle scalene will help elevate the first rib during forced inhalation. The posterior scalene will help elevate the second rib during forced inhalation.* [3 p.793] It is common to have a tender point in one of the scalenes (posterior to the clavicle at the base of the neck) with a first or second inhalation rib dysfunction.

C. Ligaments

The *alar* ligament extends from the sides of the dens to the lateral margins of the foramen magnum. The *transverse* ligament of the atlas attaches to the lateral masses of C1 to hold the dens in place. Rupture of this ligament (which may occur with rheumatoid arthritis) will result in catastrophic neurological damage. [1 p.541]

D. Nerves

There are 8 cervical nerve roots (see fig 2.2). *The upper seven exit above their corresponding vertebrae.* For example, the C7 nerve root will exit between C6 and C7. The last cervical nerve root (C8) will exit between C7 and T1. The brachial plexus is made up of nerve roots from C5 - T1, therefore damage to the lower cervical cord will cause neurological symptoms in the upper extremity.

Fig 2.2: Nerve roots in the cervical region will exit above the corresponding vertebrae.

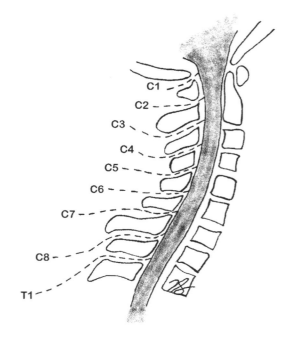

II. Motion and mechanics

Important:
Cervical spine mechanics DO NOT follow Fryette's principles I and II

A. OA - The OA is considered to be the occipital motion on the atlas (C1). *Its primary motion is flexion and extension. Sidebending and rotation occur to opposite sides.* Therefore, if the OA is sidebent left and rotated right, then it means that the occiput on the atlas is sidebent left and rotated right.

B. AA- The AA is considered to be C1 motion on C2. *Its primary motion is rotation* (50% of the rotation of the cervical spine occurs here). *Sidebending and rotation occur to opposite sides.* Therefore, if the AA is rotated right and sidebent left, then it means that the atlas (C1) is rotated right and sidebent left on the axis (C2).

C. C2-C7- *Sidebending and rotation occur to the same side. The primary motion for the upper cervicals is rotation. The primary motion for the lower cervicals is sidebending.*

Table 2.1

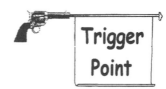

Segment	Main motion	Rotation and Sidebending
OA	Flexion and Extension	Opposite sides
AA	Rotation	Opposite sides
Upper cervical	Rotation	Same sides
Lower cervical	Sidebending	Same sides

D. Motion testing

1. Translation- (best for evaluation of the OA). Right translation will induce left sidebending. Therefore, if the OA is restricted in right translation in the flexed position, it suggests an occiput that is extended, rotated left and sidebent right (i.e., restriction of flexion, rotating right and sidebending left).

Right Translation = Force from Right to Left = Left Sidebending

2. <u>Rotation</u>- (best for evaluation of the AA). To test the AA for rotational somatic dysfunction, *remember to flex the neck to 45⁰ to lock out C2-C7*. A right rotated atlas exhibits restriction in left rotation. Osteopathic terminology for this dysfunction is *posterior atlas right.* [1 p.544]

3. <u>C2-C7-</u> are typically evaluated using translation. A translatory force is directed at the articular pillars to induce sidebending.

III. <u>Important considerations about the cervical spine</u>

1. Suboccipital or paravertebral muscle spasms are usually associated with upper thoracic or rib problems on the same side. Therefore, treat these areas first, then treat the cervical spine. [1 p.545]

2. An acute injury to the cervical spine is best treated with indirect fascial techniques or counterstrain first. [1 p.545]

Chapter **3**
Thorax and Ribcage

Thorax

I. Anatomy
A. Rule of three's
Spinous processes are large and point increasingly downward from T1-T9, then back to almost an anterior-posterior orientation from T10-T12. [1 p.563] A useful way to identify the thoracic transverse processes from the location of the corresponding spinous process involves the "**rule of three's**":

1. T1-T3 - the transverse process is *located at the level of the corresponding spinous process.*
2. T4-T6 - the transverse process is locate one-half a segment above the corresponding spinous *process.* For example, the transverse process of T5 is located halfway between the spinous processes of T4 and T5.
3. T7-T9 - the transverse process is located at the level of *the spinous process of the vertebrae above.* For example, the transverse process of T8 is at the level of T7's spinous process.
4. T10-T12 is as follows:
    T10 follows the same rules as T7-T9.
    T11 follows the same rules as T4-T6.
    T12 follows the same rules as T1-T3.

B. Other anatomical landmarks

◊ The spine of the scapula corresponds with T3.
◊ The inferior angle of the scapula corresponds with T7.
◊ The sternal notch is level with T2.
◊ The sternal angle (angle of Louis) attaches to the 2nd rib and level with T4.
◊ The nipple is at the T4 dermatome.
◊ The umbilicus is at the T10 dermatome.

II. Thoracic motion

A. *The main motion of the thorax is rotation.* However, some authors suggest that lower segment (T11 and T12) motion is similar to that of the lumbar region.
These authors report the following: [1 p.572]
◊ Upper and middle thoracic: Rotation > flexion/extension > sidebending.
◊ Lower thoracic: Flexion/extension > sidebending > rotation.

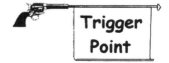

Trigger Point

Main motion of the thoracic spine = Rotation

III. Muscles of Respiration
A. Primary muscles
1. Diaphragm
Action:
  a. contracts with inspiration.
  b. causes pressure gradients to help return lymph and venous blood back to the thorax.
Attachments: xyphoid process, ribs 6-12 on either side, and bodies and intervertebral discs of L1-L3.
Innervation: Phrenic nerve (C3-C5).

2. Intercostals (external, internal, innermost, and subcostal)
Action:
a. elevate ribs during inspiration
b. prevent retractions during inspiration

B. Secondary muscles
◊   scalenes
◊   pectoralis minor
◊   serratus anterior and posterior
◊   quadratus lumborum
◊   latissimus dorsi

Ribcage
I. Anatomy
A. Typical vs. Atypical ribs
What makes a typical rib typical?
A typical rib will have all of the following anatomical landmarks:
1. Tubercle- *articulates with the corresponding transverse process.*
2. Head- *articulates with the vertebra above and corresponding vertebra.*
3. Neck
4. Angle
5. Shaft

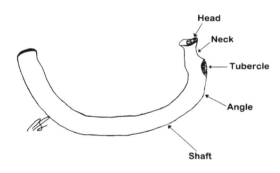

Fig 3.1: Typical rib

Typical ribs: 3-10
Atypical ribs: 1,2,11 and 12
NOTE: Sometimes rib 10 is considered atypical.
◊   Rib 1 - atypical because it articulates only with T1 and has no angle.
◊   Rib 2 - atypical because it has a large tuberosity on the shaft for the serratus anterior.
◊   Rib 11 and 12 - atypical because they articulate only with the corresponding vertebrae and lack tubercles.
◊   Rib 10 - sometimes considered atypical because it articulates only with T10.

B. True, False and Floating ribs
1. Ribs 1-7 attach directly or through chondral masses to the sternum, therefore are called **TRUE ribs.**
2. Ribs 8-10 do not directly connect to the sternum, therefore are called **FALSE ribs.**
3. Ribs 11-12 do not connect to the sternum at all, therefore are called **FLOATING ribs.**

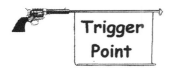

Trigger Point — Know the difference between true, floating and false ribs.

II. Rib motion

There are three classifications of rib movement:
1. Pump-handle motion
2. Bucket-handle motion
3. Caliper motion

<u>NOTE</u>: All ribs have a varying proportion of these motions depending on their location within the ribcage.

◊ *The upper ribs (ribs 1-5) move **primarily** in a pump-handle motion.*
◊ *The middle ribs (ribs 6-10) move **primarily** in a bucket-handle motion.*
◊ *The lower ribs (ribs 11 and 12) move **primarily** in a caliper motion.*

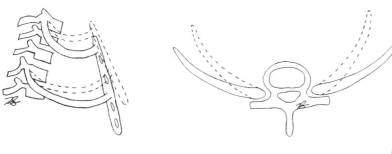

Fig 3.2a: (left) Pump-handle movement of ribs 1-5. The dotted lines show rib position in inhalation.
Fig 3.2b: (right) Caliper motion of floating ribs. The dotted lines represent rib position in exhalation.

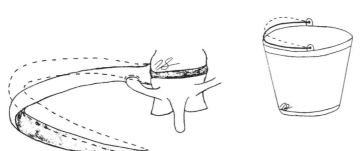

Fig 3.2c: Bucket-handle movement. A posterior-anterior view of a mid-thoracic rib. Note, that with inspiration, the rib moves up, similar to a bucket-handle

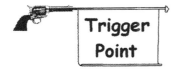

Trigger Point — Know the three different classifications of rib movement.

III. Rib dysfunctions:

A. Inhalation dysfunction (older terminology: exhalation restriction)
◊ Rib or a group of ribs will be "stuck up".

B. Exhalation dysfunction (older terminology: inhalation restriction)
◊ Rib or a group of ribs will be "stuck down".

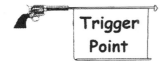

Trigger Point — Know the difference between inhalation and exhalation rib dysfunctions.

NOTE: <u>**Group dysfunctions**</u>

In these cases, there is usually one rib that is responsible in causing the dysfunction. This rib is referred to as the "key" rib.

◊   *In inhalation dysfunctions the key rib is the lowest rib of the dysfunction.*

◊   *In exhalation dysfunctions the key rib is the uppermost rib of the dysfunction.*

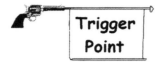

Trigger Point

Know the "key" rib in group somatic dysfunctions.

Chapter 4
Lumbar Spine

I. Anatomy

A. Important clinical points

There are five lumbar vertebrae distinguishable by their large quadrangular spinous processes. The large cross-sectional area of the lumbar vertebral body is designed to sustain longitudinal loads. [1 p.582]

The posterior longitudinal ligament runs vertically along the posterior aspect of the vertebral body. *This ligament begins to narrow at the lumbar region.* At L4 and L5 the posterior longitudinal ligament is one-half the width of that at L1. This narrowing produces a weakness in the posteriolateral aspect of the intervertebral disc. *This weakness makes the lumbar spine more susceptible to disc herniations.*

In the thoracic and lumbar region a *nerve root will exit the intervertebral foramen __below__ its corresponding segment (see fig 4.1).* For example, the L4 nerve root will exit the spinal column between L4 and L5. The spinal cord usually terminates between L1 and L2. Therefore, the exiting nerve roots become longer as they approach the lower segments, causing the *lumbar nerve roots to exit the superior aspect of their corresponding intervertebral foramina, just __above__ the intervertebral disc.* This information is important when considering disc herniations (discussed later).

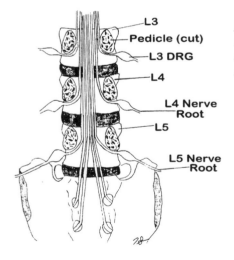

L3
Pedicle (cut)
L3 DRG
L4
L4 Nerve Root
L5
L5 Nerve Root

Fig 4.1: (DRG = Dorsal Root Ganglion) Lumbar nerve roots exit intervertebral foramen below the corresponding segment, but above the intervertebral disc.

B. Muscles

◊ Erector spinae group (spinalis, longissimus, iliocostalis)
◊ Multifidus and rotatores
◊ Quadratus lumborum
◊ Iliopsoas - composed of the psoas major muscle and iliacus muscle. *The iliopsoas is the primary flexor of the hip.* Somatic dysfunction of the iliopsoas muscle is very common, and is usually precipitated from prolonged shortening of the muscle. *An exaggerated lumbar lordosis, a positive Thomas test, and somatic dysfunction of the upper lumbar segments is commonly seen with iliopsoas dysfunctions* (for further discussion see flexion contracture of the iliopsoas). The iliopsoas also plays an important role in maintaining the lumbosacral angle.

C. Anatomical landmarks
◊   L4 - L5 intervertebral disc at the level of the iliac crest.
◊   T10 dermatome at the umbilicus, which is anterior to L3 and L4 intervertebral disc.

D. Anatomical variations
1. Sacralization- a bony deformity in which one or both of the transverse processes of L5 are long and articulate with the sacrum. Sacralization is present in 3.5% of individuals, [4 p.367] and may alter the structure-function relationship of the lumbosacral junction, leading to early disc degeneration.

2. Lumbarization- results from the failure of fusion of S1 with the other sacral segments. Lumbarization is much less common than sacralization.

3. Spina Bifida- a developmental anomaly in which there is a defect in the closure of the lamina of the vertebral segment. It usually occurs in the lumbar spine. There are three types of spinal bifida:
   a. **Spina Bifida meningocele** - A herniation of the meninges through the defect.
   b. **Spina Bifida meningomyelocele** - A herniation of the meninges and the nerve roots through the defect.
   c. **Spina Bifida occulta** - No herniation through the defect. Often the only physical sign of this anomaly is a course patch of hair over the site.

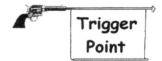
Trigger Point   **Know definition and different types of Spina Bifida.**

II. Lumbar mechanics and Somatic dysfunction
Due to the alignment of the facets (backward and medial for the superior facets), *the major motion of the lumbar spine is flexion and extension.* There is a small degree of sidebending and a very limited amount of rotation. Motion of the lumbar spine will follow Fryette's principles. Somatic dysfunction may occur in any of the three planes of motion.

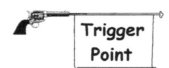
Trigger Point   **Main motion of the lumbar spine = Flexion/Extension.**

A. Motion of the L5 will influence the motion of the sacrum in two ways:
1. Sidebending of L5 will cause a sacral oblique axis to be engaged on the same side.
2. Rotation of the L5 will cause the sacrum to rotate toward the opposite side.

For a further description of the influence of L5 on lumbosacral mechanics, see Chapter 5 Sacrum and Innominates.

Copyright 1999

III. Lumbosacral angle (Ferguson's angle) (see fig 4.3)

The lumbosacral angle is formed by the intersection of a horizontal line and the line of inclination of the sacrum. This angle is normally between 25° and 35°. [2 p.164] An increase in Ferguson's angle causes a shear stress placed on the lumbosacral joint, often causing low back pain.

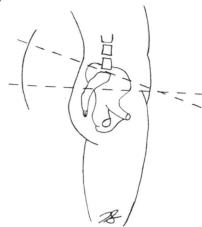

Fig 4.3: Ferguson's angle: The angle formed between the two dotted lines (normally 25° - 35°).

IV. Common problems that cause low back pain

Low back pain may be acute or chronic. Acute causes of low back pain may be due to fracture, recent strain or disc herniation, an infection, such as osteomyelitis or meningitis, or it may be referred pain. Chronic causes of low back pain are much more common. It is important as a physician to distinguish between congenital, metabolic, neoplastic, and degenerative cause of low back pain. Since there are several causes of low back pain, our discussion will be limited to the mechanical causes of low back pain. Although not very common, another important cause of low back pain is cauda equina syndrome, which will also be discussed.

A. Somatic dysfunctions of the lumbosacral spine (back strain)

◊ Location of back pain: low back, buttock, posterior lateral thigh. [7 p.183]
◊ Quality of pain: ache, muscle spasm. [7 p.183]
◊ Signs and Symptoms: increased pain with activity or prolonged standing or sitting, increased muscle tension.
◊ Treatment: OMT consisting of counterstrain for tenderpoints, muscle energy or HVLA for restrictions. OMT should also be directed at decreasing restrictions in other areas that may alter the structure-function relationship of the lumbosacral spine.

B. Herniated nucleus pulposus

◊ Pathogenesis: Due to the narrowing of the posterior longitudinal ligament, a posteriolateral herniation of the intervertebral disc is a common problem. Ninety-eight percent of herniations occur between L4 and L5, or between L5 and S1. [7 p.191] *A herniated disc in the lumbar region will exert pressure on the nerve root of the vertebrae below* . For example, a herniation between L5 and S1 will affect the nerve root of S1 (see fig 4.1).
◊ Location of pain: lower back and lower leg.
◊ Quality of pain: sharp, burning and/or shooting pain radiating down the leg, which worsens with flexion of the lumbar spine.
◊ Signs and Symptoms: weakness and decreased reflexes associated with that nerve root. Sensory deficit over the corresponding dermatome. Positive straight leg raising test.
◊ Radiology: MRI is the gold standard.
◊ Treatment: less than 5% are surgical candidates. Most cases can be treated conservatively with bed rest initially, then OMT to help decrease restrictions and improve the structure-function relationship of the lumbosacral spine.

C. Flexion contracture of the iliopsoas

◊   <u>Pathogenesis</u>: often precipitated from prolonged positions that shorten the psoas. [1] *p.597*

◊   <u>Location of pain</u>: low back sometimes radiating to groin.

◊   <u>Quality of pain</u>: ache, muscle spasm.

◊   <u>Signs and symptoms</u>: increased pain when standing or walking, positive Thomas test, tender point medial to ASIS, *nonneutral dysfunction of L1 or L2.*

◊   <u>Treatment</u>: OMT should be directed at decreasing the muscle spasm (counterstrain), and treating the nonneutral dysfunction if present.

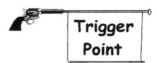

Trigger Point

A flexion contracture of the iliopsoas is often associated with a nonneutral dysfunction of L1 or L2.

D. Spinal stenosis

◊   <u>Definition</u>: Narrowing of the spinal canal, causing pressure on the roots (or rarely the cord) prior to their exit from the foramina. [8] *p.1363*

◊   <u>Pathogenesis</u>: With osteoarthrosis (the most common form), degenerative changes occur in the facet joints in association with alterations in intervertebral disc, and soft tissue structures decrease the size of the spinal canal. [7] *p.198*

◊   <u>Location of pain</u>: low back to lower leg.

◊   <u>Quality of pain</u>: ache, shooting pain or parasthesias.

◊   <u>Signs and symptoms</u>: pain with standing and walking.

◊   <u>Radiology</u>: osteophytes and decreased intervertebral disc space is usually present.

◊   <u>Treatment</u>: NSAIDs and lumbar braces in most cases. OMT should be directed at decreasing any restrictions or asymmetry, and correcting any muscular imbalance that are often associated with symptomatic spinal stenosis.

E. Spondylolisthesis (see fig 4.4)

◊   <u>Definition</u>: *anterior displacement* of one vertebrae in relation to the one below. [1] *p.1138* Often occurs to L4 or L5, and is usually due to fatigue fractures in the pars interarticularis of the vertebrae.

◊   <u>Location of pain</u>: low back, posterior thigh, lower leg.

◊   <u>Quality of pain</u>: ache.

◊   <u>Signs and symptoms</u>: increased pain with activity.

◊   <u>Radiology</u>: forward displacement and defect present.

◊   <u>Treatment</u>: most patients can be managed with controlled activity, mild analgesics or a lumbar brace.

F. Spondylolysis (see fig 4.5) - a defect **without** anterior displacement of the vertebral body is absent. Symptoms are similar to spondylolisthesis, and treatment is the same. **Radiographically, the fracture in the pars interarticularis is often described as a "collar" on the scotty dog.**

G. Spondylosis (see fig 4.6) - degenerative changes within the intervertebral disc and ankylosing of adjacent vertebral bodies. [1] *p.1138*

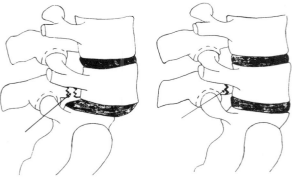

Fig 4.4: Spondylolistheis (left): The arrow
   shows a fracture of the pars interarticularis
   with anterior displacement of L5 on the
   sacrum
Fig 4.5 Spondylolysis (right): The arrow shows
   a fracture of the pars interarticularis without
   anterior displacement.

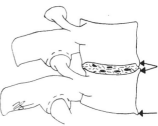

Fig 4.6: Spondylosis: Three arrows show the anterior lipping of the
   vertebral bodies. Note the associated degenerative changes within the
   intervertebral disc.

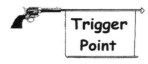

Trigger Point

> **Know the difference between spondylolisthesis, spondylolysis, and spondylosis.**

H. Cauda Equina Syndrome [7 p.682, 9 p.481]
   ◊   Definition: pressure on the nerve roots of the cauda equina usually due to a massive central disc herniation.
   ◊   Location of pain: low back.
   ◊   Quality of pain: sharp.
   ◊   Signs and symptoms: Saddle anesthesia, decreased deep tendon reflexes, decreased rectal tone, and loss of bowel and bladder control.
   ◊   Treatment: Emergent surgical decompression of the cauda equina is imperative. If surgery is delayed too long, irreversible paralysis may result.

Chapter 5
Sacrum & Innominates

I. Anatomy

A. Bones and bony landmarks

The innominate is composed of three fused bones. The ilium, the ishium and pubis bones are partially cartilaginous at birth and eventually fuse by age twenty. [1 p.601] The sacrum is composed of five fused vertebrae. The anterior portion of the first segment (S1) is referred to as the sacral promontory. The sacrum contains four bilateral foramen lateral to the sacral tubercles (sacral spinous processes). Dorsal and ventral rami from sacral nerves pass through these foramina.

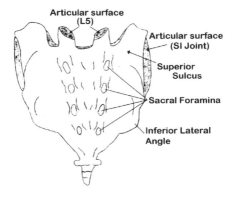

Fig 5.1: The sacrum

Articular surface (L5)
Articular surface (SI Joint)
Superior Sulcus
Sacral Foramina
Inferior Lateral Angle

B. Articulations

The innominates articulate with the femur at the acetabulum, the sacrum at the SI joint, and the pubic bones articulate with each other at the pubic symphysis. The SI joint is an "L" shaped joint with upper and lower arms. These two arms join at S2. Somatic dysfunction may occur in one or both arms of the SI joint. [1 p. 619]

C. Ligaments

1. Sacrotuberous ligament - originates at the sacrum and attaches to the ischial tuberosity.
2. Sacrospinous ligament - originates at the sacrum and attaches to the ischial spines. *This ligament divides the greater and lesser sciatic foramen.*
3. Sacroiliac ligaments - three ligaments surrounding the SI joint. Anterior, posterior and interosseous sacroiliac ligaments help stabilize the SI joint.

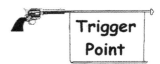

Trigger Point

The Sacrospinous ligament divides the greater and lesser sciatic foramen.

D. Muscles
1. Pelvic diaphragm - composed of the levator ani and coccygeus muscles.
2. Piriformis
   ◊ Origin - at the inferior anterior aspect of the sacrum.
   ◊ Insertion - the greater trochanter of the femur.
   ◊ Action - externally rotates, extends thigh and abducts thigh with hip flexed.
   ◊ Innervation - S1 & S2 nerve roots.
   ◊ **Clinical importance** - approximately 11% of the population will have either the entire or peroneal portion of the sciatic nerve running through the belly of the piriformis. Therefore, piriformis hypertonicity can cause buttock pain that radiates down the thigh, but not usually below the knee. This is more commonly known as sciatica. [1 p.605]

II. Sacral and innominate mechanics
A. Innominates
Physiologically, the innominates rotate about an inferior transverse axis of the sacrum. However, during dysfunctions there may be multiple axes of rotation.

B. Sacrum
1. **Four types of sacral motion** (see fig 5.2)
   a. Postural motion- *Motion occurs about the transverse axis through S3.* The sacral base will move posterior with forward bending. The sacral base will move anterior with backward bending. [1 p.607]
   b. Respiratory motion- *Motion occurs about a transverse axis through S2.* During inhalation, the sacral base will move posterior. During exhalation, the sacral base will move anterior. [1 p.607]
   c. Inherent motion- *Motion occurs about a transverse axis through S2* (same axis for respiratory motion). *During craniosacral flexion, the sacrum extends or **counternutates**. During craniosacral extension, the sacrum flexes or **nutates**.* [1 p.607-8] Nutation and counternutation are new terms encouraged by the Education Council on Osteopathic Principles to describe sacral movement in the cranial cycle of flexion and extension.
   d. Dynamic motion- *Motion that occurs during ambulation.* As weight bearing shifts from one side to the other while walking, the sacrum engages two sacral oblique axes. *Weight bearing on the left leg (stepping forward with the right leg) will cause a left sacral axis to be engaged.* The opposite is true for weight bearing on the right leg. [1 p.608]

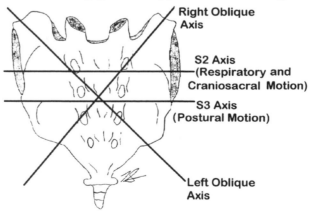

Right Oblique Axis

S2 Axis (Respiratory and Craniosacral Motion)

S3 Axis (Postural Motion)

Left Oblique Axis

Fig 5.2: Physiologic axes of the sacrum: Respiratory and Craniosacral motions occurs about a transverse axis at S2. Postural motion occurs about a transverse axis at S3. Dynamic motion occurs about a left or right oblique axes.

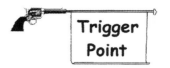

Know the physiologic motion and axes of the sacrum.

2. **Rules of L5 on the Sacrum**
    a. **Rule #1**: *When L5 is sidebent, a sacral oblique axis is engaged on the same side as the sidebending.*
    b. **Rule #2**: *When L5 is rotated, the sacrum rotates the opposite way on an oblique axis.*
    c. **Rule #3**: *The seated flexion test is found on the opposite side of the oblique axis.*

Putting the rules together:
    If L5 is $FR_R S_R$:
        There will be a positive seated flexion test on the left.
        The sacrum will be rotated to the left on a right oblique axis or L on R.

    If L5 is $NS_L R_R$:
        There will be a positive seated flexion test on the right.
        The sacrum will be rotated to the left on a left oblique axis or L on L.

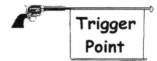

Know the rules of L5 on the sacrum.

III. Somatic dysfunctions of the innominates and sacrum
A. **Innominate dysfunction** (Remember, the side of the positive standing flexion test is the side of the dysfunction.)
    1. **Anterior innominate rotation**
       One innominate will rotate anteriorly compared to the other.
       ◊   Etiology: tight quadriceps.
       ◊   Static findings:
           ASIS more inferior ipsilaterally.
           PSIS more superior ipsilaterally.
           Longer leg ipsilaterally.
       ◊   Dynamic findings:
           AP compression restricted ipsilaterally.
           Innominate rocking restricted (resistance to posterior rotation) ipsilaterally.
           Positive standing flexion test ipsilaterally.

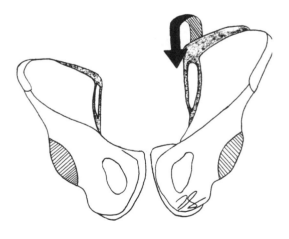

Fig 5.3: Left innominate anterior

2. **Posterior innominate rotation**
   One innominate will rotate posteriorly compared to the other.
   ◊ Etiology: tight hamstrings.
   ◊ Static findings:
      ASIS more superior ipsilaterally.
      PSIS more inferior ipsilaterally.
      Shorter leg ipsilaterally.
   ◊ Dynamic findings:
      AP compression restricted ipsilaterally.
      Positive standing flexion test ipsilaterally.

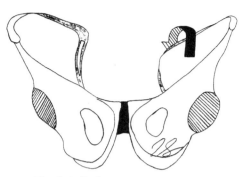

Fig 5.4: Left innominate posterior

3. **Superior innominate shear (innominate upslip, superior innominate subluxation)**
   One innominate will slip superiorly compared to the other.
   ◊ Etiology: It can be due to a fall on the ipsilateral buttock.
   ◊ Static findings:
      ASIS & PSIS more superior ipsilaterally.
      Pubic rami may be superior ipsilaterally.
   ◊ Dynamic findings:
      AP compression restricted ipsilaterally.
      Innominate rocking restricted (resistance to posterior rotation) ipsilaterally.
      Positive standing flexion test ipsilaterally.

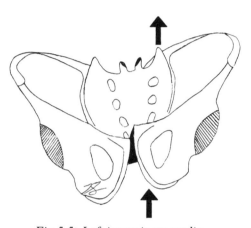

Fig 5.5: Left innominate upslip

4. **Inferior innominate shear (innominate downslip inferior innominate subluxation)**
   One innominate will slip inferiorly compared to the other.
   ◊ Static findings:
      ASIS & PSIS more inferior ipsilaterally.
      Pubic rami may be inferior ipsilaterally.
   ◊ Dynamic findings:
      AP compression restricted ipsilaterally.
      Innominate rocking restricted (resistance to posterior rotation) ipsilaterally.
      Positive standing flexion test ipsilaterally.

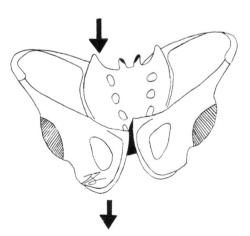

Fig 5.6 Right innominate downslip

5. **Superior pubic shear**
   A condition where one pubic bone is displaced superiorly compared to the other.
   ◊   Etiology: trauma or a tight rectus abdominus muscle.
   ◊   Static findings:
       ASIS may be level or superior ipsilaterally
       PSIS may be level or inferior ipsilaterally.
       Pubic bone superiorly ipsilaterally.
   ◊   Dynamic findings:
       Positive standing flexion test ipsilaterally.
       AP compression restricted ipsilaterally.

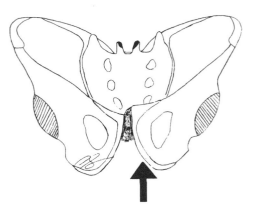

Fig 5.7: Left superior pubic shear

7. **Inferior pubic shear**
   A condition where one pubic bone is displaced inferiorly compared to the other.
   ◊   Etiology: trauma or tight adductors.
   ◊   Static findings:
       ASIS may be level or inferior ipsilaterally.
       PSIS may be level or superior ipsilaterally.
       AP compression restricted ipsilaterally.
       Pubic bone inferiorly ipsilaterally.
   ◊   Dynamic findings:
       Positive standing flexion test ipsilaterally.
       Innominate rocking restricted (resistance to posterior rotation) ipsilaterally.

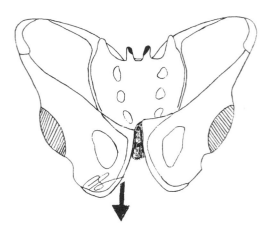

Fig 5.8: Right inferior pubic shear

8. **Innominate inflares and outflares**
   A condition where the innominate will rotate medially (inflare) or laterally (outflare).
   ◊   Static findings:
       ASIS will be more medial on an inflare.
       ASIS will be more lateral on an outflare.

B. **Sacral somatic dysfunction**
   There are two models to describe sacral dysfunction.

   1. In 1938, Strachan described sacral movements in relation to the ilium. Strachan noted two sacral somatic dysfunctions.

       a.   Anterior sacrum - the sacral base will rotate **forward** and sidebend to the opposite side of rotation.
       b.   Posterior sacrum - the sacral base will rotate **backward** and sidebend to the opposite of the rotation.

NOTE: the two somatic dysfunctions listed above is an older form for describing sacral dysfunctions. Most osteopathic institutions do not teach this model, however in order to be complete, it was included here.

2. In 1958, Miller described sacral motion in relation to L5. According to Miller, three sacral somatic dysfunctions are possible. They are:
   a. Sacral torsions
   b. Sacral shears (unilateral sacral flexions/extensions)
   c. Bilateral sacral flexions/extensions

C. Sacral Torsions

Sacral rotation about an oblique axis along with somatic dysfunction at L5. The oblique axis will run through the superior sulcus ipsilaterally, diagonally across the sacrum, through the contralateral ILA.

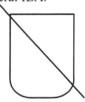

Fig 5.9: Posterior view of the sacrum with a left oblique axis.

1. Forward sacral torsion

In a forward sacral torsion, rotation is on the same side of the axis.
Two dysfunctions are possible:

a. Left rotation on a left oblique axis (L on L): left rotation occurs as the right superior sulcus moves anterior while the left ILA moves posterior.
   ◊ Static findings:
     Right superior sulcus deeper.
     Left ILA shallow.
     Lumbar curve convex to the right.
   ◊ Dynamic findings:
     Positive seated flexion test on the RIGHT.
     Restricted springing on the left ILA.
     L5 will be sidebent left rotated right (NS_LR_R) or sidebent toward the concavity and rotated toward the convexity.

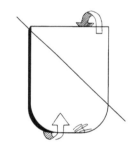

b. Right rotation on a right oblique axis (R on R): right rotation occurs as the left superior sulcus moves anterior, while the left ILA moves posterior.
   ◊ Static findings:
     Left superior sulcus deeper.
     Right ILA shallow.
     Lumbar curve convex to the left.
   ◊ Dynamic findings:
     Positive seated flexion test on the LEFT.
     Restricted springing on the right ILA.
     L5 will be sidebent right, rotated left (NS_RR_L), or sidebent toward the concavity, rotated toward the convexity.

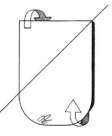

2. **Backward sacral torsion**

In a backward sacral torsion rotation is on the opposite side of the axis.

Two dysfunctions are possible:

a. <u>Right rotation on a left oblique axis (R on L)</u>: right rotation occurs as the right superior sulcus moves posterior, and the left ILA moves anterior.

◊ <u>Static findings</u>:
Right superior sulcus shallow.
Left ILA deeper.
Lumbar curve convex to the right.

◊ <u>Dynamic findings</u>:
Positive seated flexion test on the RIGHT.
Positive lumbosacral spring test.
Positive backward bending test.
Restricted springing on the right superior sulcus.
L5 will be flexed or extended (nonneutral), sidebent left, rotated left (NNR_LS_L), or sidebent and rotated toward the concavity.

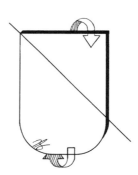

b. <u>Left rotation on a right oblique axis (L on R)</u>: left rotation occurs as the left superior sulcus moves posterior, and the right ILA moves anterior.

◊ <u>Static findings</u>:
Left superior sulcus shallow.
Right ILA deeper.
Lumbar curve convex to the left.

◊ <u>Dynamic findings</u>:
Positive seated flexion test on the LEFT.
Positive lumbosacral spring test.
Positive backward bending test.
Restricted springing on the left superior sulcus.
L5 will be flexed or extended (nonneutral), sidebent right, rotated right (NNR_RS_R), or sidebent and rotated toward the concavity.

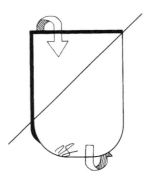

D. **Bilateral sacral flexion and extension**

1. <u>Bilateral sacral flexion (sacral base anterior)</u> [1. P.620-1]

In this somatic dysfunction, the entire sacral base moves anterior.

◊ <u>Static findings</u>:
Right and left superior sulci deep.
Increased lumbar curve.
ILA's shallow bilaterally.

◊ <u>Dynamic findings</u>:
Negative lumbosacral spring test. [1 p.615]
Restricted springing on ILA's bilaterally.
FALSE negative seated flexion test.
<u>NOTE</u>: since both SI joints are restricted in this dysfunction, asymmetry cannot be appreciated, resulting in a false negative seated and standing flexion tests.

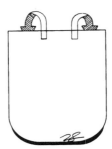

2. Bilateral sacral extensions (sacral base posterior)
In this somatic dysfunction, the entire sacral base moves posterior.
◊   Static findings:
Right and left superior sulci shallow.
Decreased lumbar curve.
ILA's deeper bilaterally.
◊   Dynamic findings:
Positive lumbosacral spring test. [1 p.615]
Restricted springing on superior sulci bilaterally.
FALSE negative seated flexion test.
NOTE: since both SI joints are restricted in this
dysfunction, asymmetry cannot be appreciated. resulting
in a false negative seated and standing flexion tests.

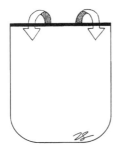

E. Sacral shears (unilateral sacral flexion/extension (USF/USE) -
In this somatic dysfunction, the sacrum will shift anteriorly or posteriorly around a transverse
axis. [1 p.621]

1. In a unilateral sacral flexion on the right (USF$_R$), the sacral base will shift anterior on the
right.
This will result in:
◊   Static findings:
Right superior sulcus deeper.
Right ILA inferior and shallow.
◊   Dynamic findings:
Positive seated flexion test on right.
Restricted springing on the right ILA.

2. In a unilateral sacral extension on the right (USE$_R$), the sacral base will shift posterior on
the right.
This will result in:
◊   Static findings:
Right superior sulcus shallow.
Right ILA superior and deeper.
◊   Dynamic findings:
Positive seated flexion test on right.
Restricted springing on the right superior pole.
Positive lumbosacral spring test.
Positive backward bending test.

F. Sacral margin posterior
Some authors do not recognize this as a true somatic dysfunction, hence there is controversy on
whether it exists. However, it is mentioned here because this dysfunction is taught at some
osteopathic institutions.

1. In a **right sacral margin posterior,** the sacrum rotates posteriorly about a vertical axis
through the opposite SI joint.

◊   Static findings:
Right superior sulci and right ILA's shallow.
◊   Dynamic findings:
Positive seated flexion test on right.
Restrictive springing on the right superior sulcus and right ILA .

IV. Clinical pearls of innominate and sacral dysfunctions

◊   As mentioned earlier, Mitchell described sacral motion in relation to L5. If a somatic dysfunction occurs in L5, a sacral somatic dysfunction is likely to be present. Therefore, if a physician uncovers a sacral somatic dysfunction, he/she should check L5 for restriction. If restriction is present then treatment should be directed toward L5 first. Most of the time the sacral dysfunction will spontaneously resolve with treatment of L5. [1] p. 622

◊   A flexion contracture of the iliopsoas may cause L1 or L2 to be flexed, sidebent, and rotated to the same side of the iliopsoas contracture. For example, if a person has a flexion contracture of the iliopsoas on the right, L1 or L2 may be FR_RS_R. [1] p.597

Chapter **6**
Upper Extremities

Shoulder
I. Anatomy
A. Bones
◊ Clavicle - acts as a strut for upper limb to allow maximum freedom of motion, as well as transmit forces from the upper extremity to the axial skeleton.
◊ Scapula
◊ Humerus

B. Joints
◊ Scapulothoracic (pseudo-joint)
◊ Acromioclavicular
◊ Sternoclavicular
◊ Glenohumeral

C. Muscles
1. <u>Rotator cuff</u> - there are four rotator cuff muscles. They serve to protect the shoulder joint and give it stability by holding the head of the humerus in the glenoid fossa. [3 p.537]

mnemonic: **SITS**

S= supraspinatus - abduction of the arm especially from 60^0 to 120^0.

I= infraspinatus - external rotation of arm.

T= teres minor - external rotation of arm.

S= subscapulais - internal rotation of arm.

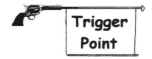

Trigger Point | **Know the rotator cuff muscles.**

2. Other muscles of the shoulder
Table 6.1 [1 p.549]

Action	Muscle
Primary flexor	Deltoid (anterior portion)
Primary abductor	Deltoid (middle portion)
Primary extensors	Latissimus dorsi, Teres major and Deltoid (posterior portion)
Primary adductors	Pectoralis major, Latissimus dorsi
Primary external rotators	Infraspinatus, Teres minor
Primary internal rotator	Subscapularis

D. Arterial supply

◊ The subclavian artery passes between the anterior and middle scalenes. The subclavian vein passes anterior to the anterior scalene. Therefore, contracture of the anterior and middle scalenes may compromise arterial supply to the arm, but not affect venous drainage.

◊ Subclavian artery becomes the axillary artery at the lateral border of the first rib.

◊ The axillary artery becomes the brachial artery at the inferior border of the teres minor muscle.

◊ The profunda brachial artery is the first major branch of the brachial artery. It accompanies the radial nerve in its posterior course of the radial groove. [3 p.547]

◊ The brachial artery divides into the ulnar and radial arteries under the bicipital aponeurosis.

◊ The radial artery courses the lateral aspect of the forearm supplying blood to the elbow, wrist, dorsal aspect of the hand, and eventually forming most of *the deep palmar arterial arch.*

◊ The ulnar artery courses the medial aspect of the forearm supplying blood to the elbow, wrist, dorsal aspect of the hand and eventually forming most of *the superficial palmar arterial arch.*

E. Lymphatic drainage of the upper extremities

◊ Right upper extremity drains into the right subclavian duct.

◊ Left upper extremity drains into the thoracic duct.

F. Nerves

The brachial plexus (fig 6.1) is responsible for supplying the nerves to the upper extremity. It is composed of nerves from roots C5-C8 and T1. A thorough neurological examination of the upper extremity demands that every physician have a good understanding of the brachial plexus.

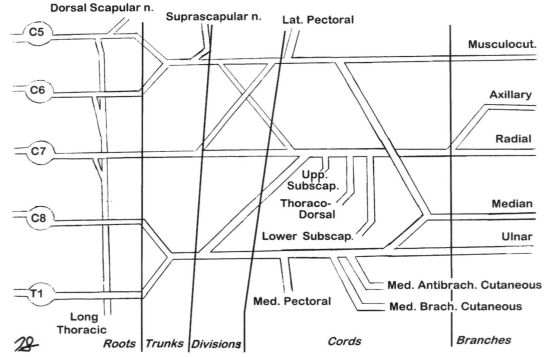

*Fig 6.1: The brachial plexus; notice how nerve **r**oots exit the spinal cord to form **t**runks which form **d**ivisions which form **C**ords which form **b**ranches. An easy mnemonic to remember this sequence is:*

Really **T**hirsty? **D**rink **C**old **B**eer!

II. Motion testing and examination of the shoulder

The four joints of the shoulder listed earlier in this chapter allow for several different motions. A restriction may develop in any of these motions. One of the more common restrictions of shoulder movement involves abduction. Normally, the arm can abduct to 180^0 with active motion, 120^0 is due to glenohumeral motion and 60^0 is due to scapulothoracic motion. *Therefore, for every 3^0 of abduction, the glenohumeral joint moves 2^0 and the scapulothoracic joint moves 1^0.* [1 p.548] A careful history and examination will reveal to the physician which joint has a restriction.

A. Motion testing of the shoulder

A good screening examination for gross range of motion of the shoulder is Apley's Scratch test. The Spencer techniques can more accurately tests individual motions of the shoulder (see Chapter 15 Articulatory Techniques). This modality can be expanded to include treatment as well.

B. Neurological examination of the upper extremity

In general, a neurological exam will consist of muscle strength, sensation, and reflex *testing.*

1. **Peripheral nerve distribution in the upper extremity** - Table 6.2 will help the examiner understand the nerve root system for the upper extremity.

Table 6.2 [5 p.57,104,149,185, 6 p.119]

Nerve root	Sensation	Motor	Reflex
C1	vertex of skull	none	none
C2	temple and occipital areas	none	none
C3	supraclavicular fossa	none	none
C4	superior aspect of shoulder	none	none
C5	lateral arm and lateral aspect of elbow	deltoid and biceps	biceps reflex
C6	lateral forearm and thumb	biceps and wrist extensors	brachioradialis reflex
C7	middle finger	triceps and wrist flexors	triceps reflex
C8	little finger and medial forearm	wrist flexors and interossi	none
T1	medial elbow and medial arm	interossi	none

2. Deep tendon reflex evaluation

Although differences may be subtle, table 6.3 shows the standard way to record the amplitude of a reflex. [1 p.552]

Table 6.3

Grade	Definition
4/4	Brisk with sustained clonus
3/4	Brisk with unsustained clonus
2/4	Normal
1/4	Decreased but present
0/4	Absent

3. Muscle strength recording

Table 6.4 shows the standard method for recording motor strength

Table 6.4 [1 p.552]

Grade	Diagnosis	Definition
5	Normal	Full range of motion (FROM) against gravity and full resistance
4	Good	FROM against gravity with some resistance
3	Fair	FROM against gravity with no resistance
2	Poor	FROM with gravity eliminated
1	Trace	Evidence of slight contractility
0	Zero	No evidence of contractility

III. Common problems of the shoulder
A. Thoracic outlet syndrome
◊   Pathogenesis: Compression of the neurovascular bundle (subclavian artery and vein, and the brachial plexus).

Compression can occur in three places: [1 p.542]
1. *Between the anterior and middle scalenes.*
2. *Between the clavicle and the first rib.*
3. *Between pectoralis minor and the upper ribs.*

Compression may be due to:
1. a cervical rib
2. excessive tension of the anterior or middle scalenes
3. somatic dysfunction of the clavicle or upper ribs
4. abnormal insertion of pectoralis minor

◊   Location of pain: Neck pain or pain radiating to arm.
◊   Quality of pain: Ache or parasthesias.
◊   Signs and Symptoms: On examination, the scalenes, a cervical rib, or the clavicle may be tender. Pulses in the upper extremity may be normal or diminished. *Often there is a positive Adson's, Roos, or Hyperabduction tests* (see Chapter 16 Special Tests).
◊   Treatment: Exercises to strengthen trapezius and levator scapula. [4 p.463] OMT should be directed at improving restriction usually found in the cervical region, upper thoracic and ribs, clavicle, scalene, and surrounding musculature. [1 p.561]

B. Supraspinatus Tendinitis
◊   Pathogenesis: Continuous impingement of the greater tuberosity against the acromion as the arm is flexed and internally rotated.
◊   Location of pain: Tenderness, especially at the top of the acromion.
◊   Signs and symptoms: It is usually a gradual onset and may be preceded by a strain. The pain is usually exacerbated by abduction, especially from 60^{0}-120^{0}. This is commonly referred to as the *"painful arc"*. *A positive drop arm test is a common sign.*
◊   Clinical manifestations: Chronic tendinitis may lead to calcification of the supraspinatus tendon.
◊   Treatment: Rest, ice and NSAIDS for the acute stages. For severe cases a sling and injection of cortisone may provide relief. OMT should be directed at the shoulder complex, upper thoracic and ribs to free up motion and loosen the fascia of the shoulder girdle to expedite the healing process.

C. Bicipital tenosynovitis
◊   Pathogenesis: An inflammation of the tendon and its sheath of the long head of the biceps. It is usually due to overuse, combined with physiological wear and tear, leading to adhesions that bind the tendon to the bicipital groove. It also may result from a subluxation of the bicepital tendon out of the bicipital groove. [1 p.559]
◊   Location of pain: Anterior portion of the shoulder which may radiate to the biceps.
◊   Signs and symptoms: Tenderness is usually present over the bicipital groove. Pain is usually aggravated by resisted flexion or supination of the forearm. [8 p. 1366]
◊   Treatment: Rest and ice for acute injury. For severe cases 2% lidocaine or cortisone may provide relief. OMT should include freeing up any restrictions in the glenohumeral area, and myofascial release.

D. Rotator cuff tear
◊ Definition: A tear at the insertion of one of the rotator cuff tendons usually the supraspinatus. Minor tears of the cuff are common. However, a complete tear can occur resulting in retraction of the affected muscle, and sharp shoulder pain.
◊ Etiology: Often associated with trauma.
◊ Location of pain: Tenderness just below the tip of the acromion.
◊ Quality of pain: A transient sharp pain in the shoulder followed by a steady ache that may last for days. [4 p.470]
◊ Signs and symptoms: In minor supraspinatus tears, a weakness in active abduction is often present along with a *positive drop arm test* (see Chapter 16 Special Tests). Atrophy is a common sign. Often the patient will experience pain for months especially at night.
◊ Treatment: For minor tears, rest, ice and NSAIDS in the acute stages. OMT should be directed at freeing up any restrictions in the glenohumeral area as well as treating the clavicle, upper thoracic, and ribs for somatic dysfunction. Surgery is required for complete avulsion.

E. Adhesive capsulitis/ Frozen shoulder syndrome
◊ Definition: A common condition characterized by pain and restriction of shoulder motion that increasingly gets worse over the course of one year.
◊ Signs and symptoms: Decreased range of motion, especially in the scapulothoracic joint. [4 p.469]
◊ Epidemiology: It is most often seen in patients over 40 years of age. [4 p.469]
◊ Etiology: *It is caused by prolonged immobility of the shoulder.*
◊ Location of pain: Tenderness is usually at the anterior portion of the shoulder.
◊ Treatment: The main goal is prevention. Early mobilization following shoulder injury is essential. Injection of corticosteriods and NSAIDS may help. OMT should be directed at improving motion and lysing adhesions. Treatment of the glenohumeral joint and upper thoracic often provide relief.

F. Shoulder dislocation (subluxation)
◊ Common in athletes and usually occurs as a result of trauma. *Humeral dislocation usually occurs anteriorly and inferiorly.* Recurrent shoulder dislocations are common and require less force.

G. Winging of the scapula
◊ *A weakness of the anterior serratus muscle usually due to a long thoracic nerve injury.* This condition is evident if the scapula protrudes posteriorly while the patient is pushing on a wall.

H. Brachial plexus injuries
◊ The nerves of the brachial plexus are susceptible to traction injury especially during childbirth. *Erb-Duchenne's palsy is by far the most common form of brachial plexus injury. It is an upper arm paralysis caused by injury to C5 and C6 nerve roots usually during childbirth.* It can result in paralysis of the deltoid, external rotators, biceps, brachioradialis, and supinator muscles. Klumpke's palsy is much less common, and is due to injury to C8 and T1. Paralysis usually occurs in the intrinsic muscles of the hand.

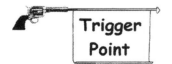
Trigger Point

Most common type of brachial plexus injury is Erb-Duchenne's palsy

Elbow, Wrist and Hand
I. **Anatomy**
A. **Bones**
     ◊   Radius
     ◊   Ulna
     ◊   Eight carpal bones

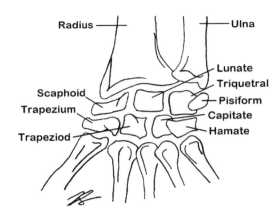

Fig 6.2: The carpal bones

MEMORY TOOL:	
Scaphoid	Some
Lunate	Lovers
Triquetral	Try
Pisiform	Positions
Trapezium	That
Trapezoid	They
Capate	Can't
Hamate	Handle

     ◊   Five metacarpals
     ◊   Fourteen phalanges

B. **Joints**
     ◊   Elbow (ulna and humerus)
     ◊   Ulna and Radial (distal and proximal)
     ◊   Intercarpals, Carpometacarpals, Metacarpophalangeal (MCP), Interphalangeal (PIP & DIP).

C. **Muscles and innervations** [1] *p.550*
     ◊   Primary **flexors of the wrist and hand** originate on or near the medial epicondyle of the humerus. Most of which are *innerveted by the median nerve* (except for flexor carpi ulnaris - ulnar nerve).

     ◊   Primary **extensors of the wrist and hand** originate at the lateral epicondyle of the humerus. All of which are *innerveted by the radial nerve.*

     ◊   Primary **supinators** of the forearm are the biceps (*musculocutaneous nerve*) and the supinator (*radial nerve*).

     ◊   Primary **pronators** of the forearm are the pronator teres and pronator quadratus (*radial nerve*).

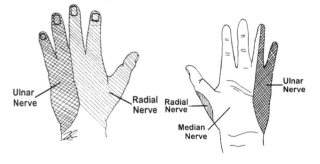

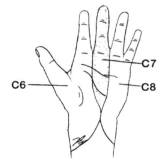

Fig 6.3: Posterior (left) and anterior (right) view of the
cutaneous distribution for the radial, ulnar, and median nerves.

Fig 6.4 (above): Anterior view of the
distribution for the nerve roots
supplying the hand

D. Muscles of the hand
◊   Muscles in the thenar eminence are innervated by the *median nerve* (except for adductor pollicis brevis - ulnar nerve).
◊   Muscles in the hypothenar eminence and interossi are innervated by the *ulnar nerve.*
◊   Lumbricles (4)
         First and Second lumbricles innervated by the *median nerve.*
         Third and Fourth lumbricles innervated by the *ulnar nerve.*

NOTE: Remember that the flexor digitorum profundus attaches to the distal interphalengeal joint (DIP). The flexor digitorum superficialis attaches to the proximal interphalangeal joint (PIP).

II. Motion of the Elbow and Forearm
A. Carrying angle (fig 6.5)
Formed by the intersection of two lines. The first line is the longitudinal axis of the humerus. The second line starts at the distal ulnar radial joint, and passes through the proximal radial ulna joint.
◊   The normal carrying angle in men is 5^0.
◊   The normal carrying angle in women is 10^0-12^0.
◊   A carrying angle $> 15^0$ is called cubitus valgus or **abduction of the ulna** if somatic dysfunction is present.
◊   A carrying angle $< 3^0$ is called cubitis varus or **adduction of the ulna** if somatic dysfunction is present.

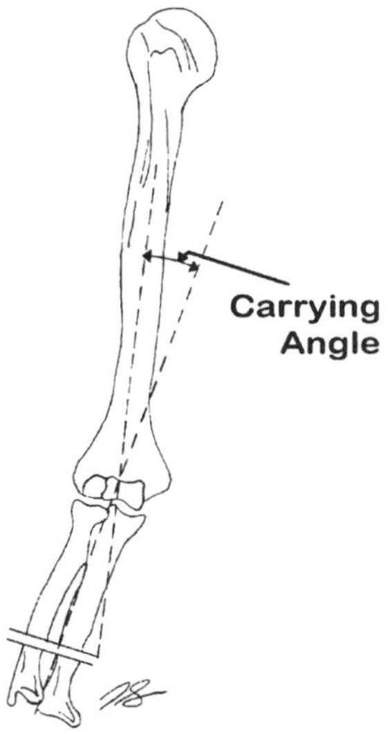

Fig 6.5: The angle formed between the two dotted lines represents the carrying angle.

◊   The carrying angle has a direct influence on the position of the wrist. Due to a parallelogram effect, **an increase in the carrying angle (abduction of the ulna) will cause an adduction of the wrist.** Conversely, **a decrease in the carrying angle (adduction of the ulna) will cause an abduction of the wrist**. [1 p.554]

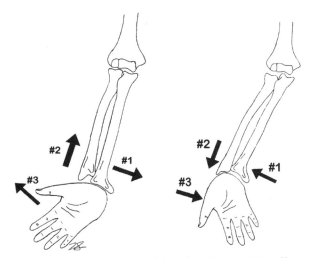

Fig 6.6 (left): Adduction of the ulna (arrow #1) will cause the radius to be pulled proximal (arrow #2). This will result in abduction of the wrist (arrow #3).
Fig 6.7 (right): Abduction of the ulna (arrow #1) will cause the radius to be pushed distal (arrow #2). This will result in adduction of the wrist (arrow #3).

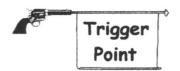

Table 6.5

Carrying Angle	Ulna Movement	Wrist Movement
Increased	Abduction	Adduction
Decreased	Adduction	Abduction

B. Radial head motion

The radial head will glide anteriorly and posteriorly with pronation and supination of the forearm.

◊ *When the forearm is pronated, the radial head will glide posteriorly.*

◊ *When the forearm is supinated, the radial head will glide anteriorly.*

III. Somatic dysfunction of the forearm

A. Abduction of the ulna

◊ Findings: the ulna will be restricted in adduction motion. *The wrist will be adducted and restricted in abduction.* See figure 6.7.

B. Adduction of the ulna

◊ Findings: the ulna will be restricted in abduction motion. *The wrist will be abducted and restricted in adduction.* See figure 6.6.

C. Posterior radial head

◊ History: Falling on a pronated forearm is often a common cause. [1 p.556]

◊ Osteopathic findings: Restricted supination of the forearm.

D. Anterior radial head

◊ History: Falling on a supinated forearm is often a common cause. [1 p.556]

◊ Osteopathic findings: Restricted pronation of the forearm.

IV. Common complaints of the wrist

A. Carpal tunnel syndrome

◊ Definition: Entrapment of the median nerve between the longitudinal tendons of the hand and the flexor retinaculum.

◊ Quality and location of pain: *The patient usually complains of parasthesias on the palmar surface of the thumb and the first 2 ½ digits.*

◊ Signs and symptoms: Weakness and atrophy usually appear late. On examination, symptoms are reproduced with *Tinel's, phalen, and prayer tests.*

◊ Treatment: Nerve conduction studies remain the gold standard for diagnosis. Treatment usually consists of splints, NSAIDS, and steroid injections. Surgery is indicated if medical treatment has failed. OMT is usually very helpful, and should be directed at correcting upper thoracic and rib dysfunctions, decreasing sympathetic tone in the upper extremity, and removing any myofascial restrictions. [1 p.560]

B. Lateral epicondylitis (tennis elbow)

◊ Definition: A strain of the extensor muscles of the forearm near the lateral epicondyle.

◊ Pathogenesis: Results from repetitive and strenuous supination, or by violent extension of the wrist with the hand pronated. [8 p.1368]

◊ Location of pain: The patient usually complains of pain over the lateral epicondyle that worsens with supination against resistance.

◊ Quality of pain: Pain may radiate to the lateral aspect of the arm and forearm.

◊ Signs and symptoms: Tenderness at the lateral epicondyle or just distal to it. Pain often worsens with activity.

◊   Treatment: NSAIDS, rest, and ice. To prevent recurrences, a four-inch strap is tightly worn around the forearm muscles during aggravating activity. [8 p.1368] OMT should be directed toward correcting cervical or upper thoracic dysfunctions, counterstrain to affected muscles (usually extensors), and myofascial release to decrease fascial restrictions.

C. Medial epicondylitis (golfer's elbow)
◊   Definition: A strain of the flexor muscles of the forearm near the medial epicondyle.
◊   Pathogenesis: Results from repetitive and strenuous pronation or by violent flexion of the wrist with the hand supinated. [8 p.1368]
◊   Location/quality of pain, signs/symptoms, treatment: Same for tennis elbow but directed at the medial epicondyle.

V. Contractures and deformities of the wrist and hand

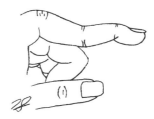

A. Swan-neck deformity (fig 6.8)
◊   Flexion contracture of the MCP and DIP.
◊   Extension contracture of the PIP.
◊   Results from a contracture of the intrinsic muscles of the hand and is often associated with *rheumatoid arthritis.*

Fig 6.8: Swan neck deformity

B. Boutonniere deformity (fig 6.9)
◊   Extension contracture of the MCP and DIP.
◊   Flexion contracture of the PIP.
◊   Results from a rupture of the hood of the extensor tendon at the PIP. It is often associated with *rheumatoid arthritis.*

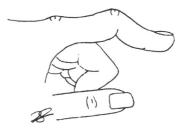

Fig 6.9: Boutonniere deformity

C. Claw hand
◊   Extension of the MCP.
◊   Flexion of the PIP and DIP.
◊   *Results from median and ulnar injury* (loss of intrinsic muscles and overactivity of the extensor muscles).

D. Ape hand
◊   Similar to the claw hand, but in addition, there is a wasting of the thenar eminence, and the thumb is adducted.
◊   *Results from median nerve damage.*

E. Bishops deformity
◊   Contracture of the last two digits with atrophy of the hypothenar eminence due to *ulnar nerve damage.*

F. Dupuytren's contracture
◊   Flexion contracture of the MCP and PIP usually seen with contracture of the last two digits. However, unlike Bishops contracture, *this is due to a contracture of the palmar fascia.*

G. Drop-wrist deformity
◊   Radial nerve damage results in paralysis of the extensor muscles

Chapter 7
Lower Extremities

Hip and Knee
I. Anatomy
A. Bones and bony landmarks
    1. <u>Femur</u> - proximally articulates with the acetabulum; distally articulates with the medial and lateral menisci that are situated on the tibial plateau.

    2. <u>Patella</u> - a sesamoid bone that attaches to the quadriceps tendon superiorly, and the patella tendon inferiorly.

    3. <u>Tibia</u>

    4. <u>Fibula</u>

B. Muscle of the hip and knee
    1. <u>Hip</u>
- ◊   Primary extensor: Gluteus maximus
- ◊   Primary flexor: Iliopsoas

    2. <u>Knee</u>
- ◊   Primary extensor: Quadriceps (rectus femoris, vastus lateralis, medialis and intermedius)
- ◊   Primary flexors: Semimembranosis and semitendinosis

C. Ligaments and joints
    1. <u>Hip</u>

      a. <u>Femoroacetabular joint (hip joint)</u> - a ball and socket joint that is held in place by the surrounding musculature and four ligaments.
- ◊   <u>Iliofemoral ligament</u>
- ◊   <u>Ishiofemoral ligament</u>
- ◊   <u>Pubofemoral ligament</u>
- ◊   <u>Capitis femoris</u> - the ligament at the head of the femur attaching to the acetabular fossa.

    2. <u>Knee</u>

The knee is composed of three joints and four major ligaments.

      a.   <u>Tibiofemoral joint</u> - the largest joint in the body. [5 p.372] The articular surfaces of the tibia and femur are separated by two "C" shaped menisci. [5 p.372] The medial and lateral menisci act as shock absorbers and also aid in nutrition and lubrication of the joint. Between the two menisci are two ligaments that help stabilize the knee.

        1)   <u>The anterior cruciate ligament (ACL)</u> - originates at the posterior aspect of the femur, and attaches to the anterior aspect of the tibia. *It prevents hyperextension of the knee.*

        2)   <u>The posterior cruciate ligament (PCL)</u> - originates on the anterior aspect of the femur and inserts on the posterior aspect of the tibia. *It prevents hyperflexion of the knee.*

b. Lateral stabilizers of the knee
    1) Medial collateral ligament (tibial collateral ligament) - originates at the femur and inserts on the tibia. This ligament also articulates with the medial meniscus.
    2) Lateral collateral ligament (fibular collateral ligament) - originates at the femur and inserts on the fibula.
c. Patellofemoral joint
d. Tibiofibular joint - a synovial joint composed of the lateral aspect of the proximal tibia and the proximal fibular head. Movement at this joint occurs with pronation and supination of the foot (figs 7.1 & 7.2).
    ◊ *The fibular head will glide anteriorly with pronation of the foot.*
    ◊ *The fibular head will glide posteriorly with supination of the foot.*

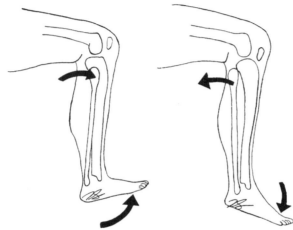

Fibular head movement:
Fig 7.1: (left) Fibular head movement. Pronation at the ankle will cause the fibular head to glide anteriorly.
Fig 7.2: (right) Supination at the ankle will cause the fibular head to glide posteriorly.

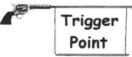

Trigger Point

1. *Dorsiflexion, eversion, and abduction = PRONATION of the ankle.* [1 p. 636]
2. *Plantarflexion, inversion and adduction = SUPINATION of the ankle.* [1 p. 636]

II. Nerves

A. Femoral nerve - (L2-L4) [6, 27]
Motor - innervates quadriceps, iliacus, sartorius and pectineus.
Sensory - anterior thigh and medial leg.

B. Sciatic nerve - (L4-S3) [6, 27] Courses through the greater sciatic foramen. In 85% of the population the sciatic nerve will be inferior to the piriformis muscle.
    Two divisions:
    1. Tibial
      a. Motor - Hamstrings except short head of the biceps femoris, most plantar flexors, and toe flexors.
      b. Sensory - Lower leg and plantar aspect of foot.

    2. Peroneal
      a. Motor - Short head of biceps femoris, evertors and dorsiflexors of the foot, and most extensors of the toes.
      b. Sensory - Lower leg and dorsum of foot.

III. Neurological evaluation

Table 7.1 [5,6]

Nerve Root	Motor	Reflex	Sensation
L1	iliopsoas	none	anterior thigh just below inguinal ligament
L2	iliopsoas, adductors, quadriceps	none	middle anterior thigh
L3	adductors, quadriceps	none	anterior thigh just above knee
L4	**anterior tibialis**	patella reflex	**medial malleolus**
L5	**ext. hallicus longus, quadriceps**	none	**dorsal aspect of foot and big toe**
S1	**peroneus longus & brevis gastrocnemius**	**achilles reflex**	**lateral malleolus**

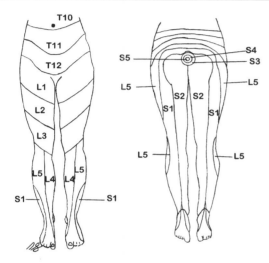

Fig 7.3: Dermatomes of the lower extremity

IV. Anatomical variations and Q angle (Quadriceps angle)

A. Angulation of the head of the femur (figs 7.4 a-c)

The normal angle between the neck and shaft of the femur is 120^0 -135^0.

*If this angle is < 120^0 this condition is called **coxa vara.**.*

*If this angle is > 135^0 this condition is called **coxa valga.***

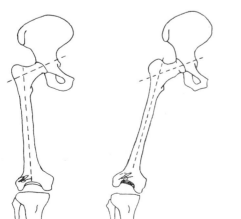
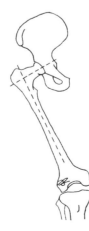

Fig 7.4a (left): Normal angle between the neck and shaft of the femur is approximately 120^0-135^0. Fig 7.4b (middle): Coxa valga; the angle between the neck and the shaft of the femur is >135^0. Fig 7.4c (right): Coxa vara; the angle between the neck and the shaft of the femur is <120^0.

B. Q angle (figs 7.5a-c)

The Q angle is formed by the intersection of a line from the ASIS through the middle of the patella, and a line from the tibial tubercle through the middle of the patella. A normal Q angle is 10^0 -12^0. [1 p.627] *An increased Q angle is referred to as genu valgum*, in which the patient will appear more knocked-kneed. *A decreased Q angle is referred to as genu varum*, in which the patient will appear more bowlegged. [1 p.627]

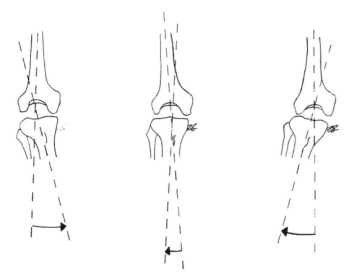

Fig 7.5a (left): Genu varum, resulting from a decreased Q angle.
Fig 7.5b (middle): Normal Q angle approximately 10^0-12^0.
Fig 7.5c (right): Genu valgum, resulting from an increased Q angle.

V. Somatic dysfunction of the fibular head

A. Fibular head dysfunction

Like all synovial joints in the body, the tibiofibular joint may develop restrictions. This may result in knee pain with activity because the fibula can bear up to 1/6 of the body weight. [5 p 374]

Two somatic dysfunctions are possible with fibular head movement:

1. **Posterior fibular head** - Present when there is a restriction in anterior glide. *The foot will appear more supinated when compared to the other side.* The fibular head will resist any anterior springing.

2. **Anterior fibular head** - Present when there is a restriction in posterior glide. *The foot will appear more pronated when compared to the other side.* The fibular head will resist any posterior springing.

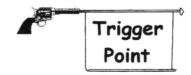

Trigger Point

The common peroneal nerve (a.k.a. common fibular nerve) lies directly posterior to the proximal fibular head. Therefore, a posterior fibular head or fracture of the fibula may disturb the function of the peroneal nerve.

VI. Clinical considerations of the hip and knee
A. Lateral femoral patella tracking syndrome
◊   Pathophysiology: An increased Q angle often causes an imbalance of the musculature of the quadriceps (strong vastus lateralis and weak vastus medialis). This imbalance will cause the patella to deviate laterally, and eventually lead to irregular or accelerated wearing on the posterior surface of the patella. [1 pp.627-8]

◊   Signs and Symptoms: Deep knee pain is present, especially when climbing stairs. The physician may notice atrophy in the vastus medialis, and often the patient will have a positive "grind test".

◊   Prevalence - Mostly in women. A wider pelvis often results in a larger Q angle.

◊   Treatment - Strengthen the vastus medialis muscle.

B. Ligamentous injury
Three grades of sprains. [1 p.623-624]
a. First degree: no tear resulting in good tensile strength and no laxity.
b. Second degree: partial tear resulting in a decreased tensile strength with mild to moderate laxity.
c. Third degree: complete tear resulting in no tensile strength and severe laxity.
NOTE: Third degree sprains may require surgery, while first and second degree sprains can be treated conservatively.

C. Compartment syndrome
Usually results from trauma or vigorous overuse leading to an increase in intracompartmental pressure. This will compromise circulation within that compartment.

The lower leg can be divided into four compartments:
1. Anterior
2. Lateral
3. Deep posterior
4. Superficial posterior
The anterior compartment is most often affected. Often resulting in severe unrelenting pain after and during exercise. The anterior tibilais muscle is hard and tender to palpation, and pulses are present, however muscles may be diminished. Treatment usually consists of ice and myofascial release, to increase venous and lymph return. If intracompartmental pressure is too great where arterial supply is reduced, a surgical fasciotomy must be done immediately. [1 p.655]

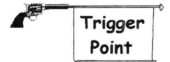
Trigger Point

O'Donahue's triad (terrible triad): a common knee injury resulting in injury to the ACL, MCL and medial meniscus.

Ankle and foot

I. Anatomy

This region consists of 26 bones articulating at 30 synovial joints, and supported by over 100 ligaments and 30 muscles.

A. Bones (fig 7.6)

◊   Talus
◊   Calcaneus
◊   Navicular
◊   Cuboid
◊   3 Cuneiforms
◊   5 Metatarsals
◊   14 Phalanges

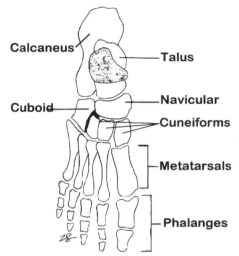

Fig 7.6: Bones of the foot: Note the gray area of the talus (the ankle mortise); it is wider anteriorly, making the foot more stable in dorsiflexion.

B. Joints

1. Talocrural joint (tibiotalar joint): a hinge joint located between the talus and the medial malleolus of the tibia, and the lateral malleolus of the fibula. [5 p.448] *The main motions of this joint are plantar flexion and dorsiflexion. Due to the configuration of the talus (the ankle mortise), the ankle is more stable in dorsiflexion than plantar flexion* (see fig. 7.6). This is the reason why 80% of ankle sprains occur in plantar flexion.

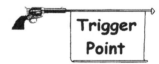

Trigger Point

The ankle is more stable in dorsiflexion.

2. Subtalar joint (talocalcaneal joint): acts mostly as a shock absorber, and also allows internal and external rotation of the leg while the foot is fixed.

C. Arches

1. Longitudinal arches:
   a. Medial longitudinal arch: talus, navicular, cuneiforms, 1st to 3rd metatarsals. [1 p.639]
   b. Lateral longitudinal arch: calcaneus, cuboid, and 4th and 5th metatarsals. [1 p.639]
2. Transverse arch: navicular, cuneiforms, and cuboid.
3. **Somatic dysfunction of the arches**

   Somatic dysfunctions usually occur within the transverse arch. The navicular, cuboid or cuneiforms may displace, causing pain. This is often seen in long distance runners.

   Three somatic dysfunctions of the transverse arch: (fig 7.7)
   a. Cuboid: the medial edge will glide toward the plantar surface.
      b. Navicular: the lateral edge will glide toward the plantar surface.
      c. Cuneiforms: usually caused by the second cuneiform gliding
         directly downward, toward the plantar surface.

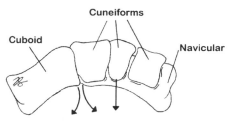

Fig 7.7: Transverse arch of the foot. It is composed of the cuboid, cuneiforms, and the navicular. Arrows show three possible somatic dysfunctions.

D. Ligaments

Since there are over one hundred ligaments in the foot and ankle, we are going to limit our discussion to the major stabilizing ligaments.

1. <u>Lateral stabilizers of the ankle</u>: These ligaments prevent excessive supination.
   a. Anterior talofibular ligament
   b. Calcaneofibular ligament
   c. Posterior talofibular ligament

Fig 7.8: Lateral stabilizers of the ankle

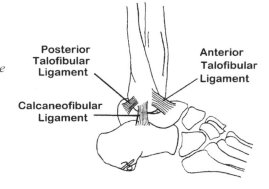

<u>Important note</u>: Due to the less stable supination position of the ankle, sprains often cause damage to these ligaments. *The most common injured ligament is the anterior talofibular ligament.* [10] *Sprains associated with the supination position are classified into 3 types depending on the extent of ligamentous injury.* [1 p.637]

Type I: involves the anterior talofibular ligament.
Type II: involves the anterior talofibular ligament and the calcaneofibular ligament.
Type III: involves the anterior talofibular ligament, calcaneofibular ligament and the posterior talofibular ligament.

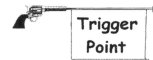

Trigger Point

> **The most common injured ligament in the foot is the Anterior Talofibular.**

2. <u>Medial stabilizers of the ankle</u>: This ligaments prevent excessive pronation.
   a. <u>Deltoid ligament</u>: Since the ankle is more stable in the pronation position and the deltoid ligament is very strong, pronation sprains are very uncommon. Excessive pronation usually result in a fracture of the medial malleolus rather than pure ligamentous injury.

3. <u>Plantar ligaments</u>
   a. <u>Spring ligament (calcaneonavicular ligament)</u>: This ligament strengthens and supports the medial longitudinal arch.
   b. <u>Plantar aponeurosis</u>: Strong, dense, connective tissue that originates at the calcaneus and attaches to the phalanges. Chronic irritation to this structure may cause calcium to be laid down along the lines of stress, leading to a heel spur. [1 p.639]

Chapter 8
Craniosacral motion

I. Introduction

The cranial field was established by William Garner Sutherland D.O. Dsci (Hon) (1873-1954). Sutherland, who graduated from the American School of Osteopathy, was an early student of A.T. Still. As a student, Sutherland noticed that the articular surfaces of the cranial bones had a unique design. After years of research and careful observations he noticed that the CNS, CSF and dural membranes functioned as a unit. He named this unit the primary respiratory mechanism (PRM). [1 p.902]

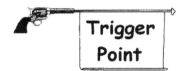

Trigger Point

CNS + CSF + Dural Membranes = PRM

The CNS, CSF and the dural membranes (PRM) function together as a physiological unit to control and regulate pulmonary respiration (which Sutherland termed *secondary respiration*), circulation, digestion. and elimination.

The PRM is composed of five anatomical-physiological elements.

       1. The inherent motility of the brain and spinal cord.
       2. Fluctuation of CSF.
       3. The mobility of the intracranial and intraspinal membranes.
       4. The articular mobility of the cranial bones.
       5. The involuntary mobility of the sacrum between the ilia.

A. The inherent motility of the brain and spinal cord
Motility vs. Mobility

If an object is motile it moves on its own; however if an object is mobile it moves only if a force acts on it.

There is much evidence in medical literature that supports cerebral motility. Four definite motions of the brain and spinal cord that have been observed during an operation: [11 p.23-4]

       1. A pulsation that is synchronous with cardiac contractions.
       2. A pulsation that coincides with pulmonary respiration.
       3. A wave not related to heart rate or respiration, but one that constantly maintains its own cycle.
       4. An undulating pulsation which has not been identified.

B. The fluctuation of the cerebral spinal fluid (CSF)

Since direct observation of the CSF would change the hydrodynamic condition under which it normally exists, experimentation is difficult. However, several authors agree that the CSF circulates with a pulsating rhythm. Hyden and others demonstrated that glial cells grown in tissue culture pulsate continuously. [11 p.24]

Sutherland discovered rhythmic impulses could be palpated on a human skull. With very gentle proprioceptive palpation, Sutherland noted that the human skull exhibited 10-14 cycles per minute. This phenomenon he called the **"Cranial Rhythmic Impulse"** or the C.R.I. [11 p.24]

C. Mobility of the intracranial and intraspinal membranes

The intracranial and intraspinal membranes (i.e. meninges), surround, support, and partition the CNS. The meninges have three membranes:

    1. Dura mater

        The dura mater is the outermost membrane. It is thick, inelastic and forms the *falx cerebri and tentorium cerebelli. The dura projects caudally down the spinal canal, with firm attachments at foramen magnum, C2, C3, and terminates at S2.*

    2. Arachnoid mater

    3. Pia mater.

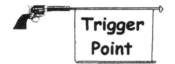

Trigger Point	**Dural attachments: Foramen magnum, C2, C3 and S2.**

The intracranial and intraspinal membranes surround support and partition the CNS. The inherent motility of the brain and spinal cord, and the fluctuation of the CSF will cause these membranes to move. Since the dura is inelastic and is attached to the cranial bones, any motion of the dura will influence the cranial bones. Therefore, the meninges will act as an inelastic rope causing the cranial bones to move in response to the motility of the brain and spinal cord, and fluctuation of the CSF. Sutherland called this "inelastic rope" the **Reciprocal Tension Membrane (RTM)**.

D. Articular mobility of the cranial bones

While Sutherland was still in medical school, he became intrigued with the articulations of the cranial sutures. The beveled surface of the sphenoid bone, and the squamous portions of the temporal bones, led Sutherland to think that articular mobility was possible. After 30 years of research on himself, and careful observation of his patients, he was convinced that the cranial bones moved in a very specific and a rhythmic type of pattern. More recently, Heisey and T. Adams demonstrated quantitatively in animal models, that cranial bones move in relation to each other. [1 p.903]

E. Involuntary mobility of the sacrum between the ilia

The inherent motility of the brain and spinal cord, and the fluctuation of CSF will cause the RTM to move. Since a portion of the RTM (the dura) *attaches to the posterior superior aspect of the second sacral segment*, any motion of the RTM will cause the sacrum to move. Research has shown that a slight rocking motion of the sacrum occurs about a *transverse axis that runs though S3. This axis is referred to as the respiratory axis.*

II. Physiologic motion of the primary respiratory mechanism

The *sphenobasilar synchondrosis* (SBS) is the articulation of the sphenoid with the occiput. It is the keystone of all cranial movement. The SBS is moved through a biphasic cycle (*flexion and extension*), in response to the pull of the dural membranes that are influenced by the coiling and uncoiling of the CNS, and the fluctuation of the CSF. [1 p.904]

A. _There are two motions that can occur at the SBS_:

1. **_Flexion_**

◊ _During flexion, the midline bones of the cranium (sphenoid, occiput, ethmoid, vomer) move through a flexion phase. The paired bones of the cranium will move through an external rotation phase._ An easy way to remember this relationship is:

During "fl **ex** ion" of midline bones,

eXternal rotation of paired bones occur.

◊ _Flexion at the SBS will cause the dura to be pulled cephalad, moving the sacral base posterior through a transverse axis about S3. This movement at the sacral base (originally termed sacral extension) is called_ **counternutation** (Fig 8.1).

◊ _Flexion will widen the head slightly and decrease its anterioposterior diameter (Fig 8.2)._

Fig 8.1 (right): Flexion of the SBS will cause the dura to be pulled cephalad, resulting in counternutation of the sacrum.

Fig 8.2 (left): Craniosacral flexion (dotted lines) will widen the head slightly and decrease the AP diameter.

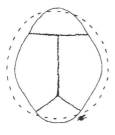

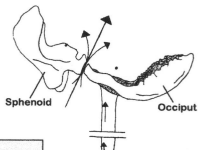

Sphenoid   Occiput

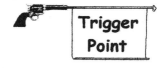

Trigger Point

Craniosacral Flexion:
1. **Flexion of midline bones.**
2. **Sacral counternutation.**
3. **Decreased AP diameter of the cranium.**

Sacral Respiratory Axis (S2)

2. **_Extension_**

◊ _During extension, the midline bones of the cranium (sphenoid, occiput, ethmoid, vomer) move through a extension phase. The paired bones of the cranium will move through an internal rotation phase._

◊ _Extension at the SBS will cause the dura to be pulled caudad, moving the sacral base anterior through a transverse axis about S3. This movement at the sacral base (originally termed sacral flexion) is called_ **nutation** (Fig 8.3).

◊ _Extension will narrow the head slightly and increase its anterioposterior diameter (Fig 8.4)._

Fig 8.3 (right): Extension of the SBS will cause the dura to be fall caudad, resulting in nutation of the sacrum.

Fig 8.4 (left): Craniosacral extension (dotted lines) will narrow the head slightly and increase the AP diameter.

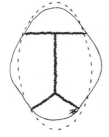

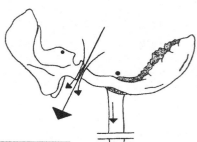

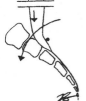

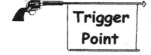

Trigger Point

Craniosacral Extension:
1. **Extension of midline bones.**
2. **Sacral nutation.**
3. **Increased AP diameter of the cranium.**

III. Strains of the sphenobasilar synchondrosis

From before birth until death, the body is subject to strains and stresses. Childbirth, traumatic brain injury, musculoskeletal dysfunction, surgery, and even everyday emotional stress are all examples of strains and stresses that may cause the PRM to be compromised. There are six types of strains that can occur at the SBS. They are: [12 p.36]

1. Flexion and extension
2. Torsion
3. Sidebending and rotation
4. Vertical strain
5. Lateral strain
6. Compression

A. Torsion

A torsion is a type of strain that occurs when there is a twisting at the SBS. *The sphenoid and other related structures of the anterior cranium rotate in one direction about an anterioposterior axis, while the occiput and the posterior cranium rotate in the opposite direction.* [1 p.906] *The torsion is named for the greater wing of the sphenoid that is more superior.* For example, if the sphenoid is rotated, so that the greater wing of the sphenoid is more superior on the right, this is called a right torsion.

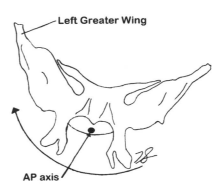

Fig 8.5: Sphenoid position in a left cranial torsion

B. Sidebending/Rotation

This type of strain has two distinct motions that occur simultaneously about three separate axes. Rotation occurs about an AP axis through the SBS (same axis as a torsion strain) (Fig 8.6b). However, unlike a torsion, in this type of strain the sphenoid and the occiput rotate in the same direction. Both bones will either rotate clockwise of counterclockwise. Sidebending occurs about two parallel vertical axes, one axis passes through foramen magnum and the other through the center of the sphenoid (Fig 8.6a). Motion will occur about these two axes so that the SBS will deviate to the right or to the left. Due to the upward convexity of the SBS, sidebending to the left (deviation of the SBS to the left) will cause the sphenoid and occiput to rotate so that they are inferior on the left. This is denoted as SBR$_L$.

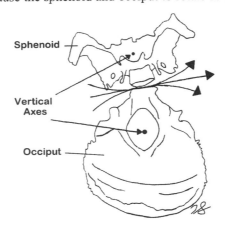

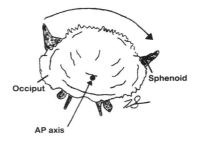

Fig 8.6a (left): Right sidebending of the SBS about two vertical axes will cause the SBS to deviate to the right.
Fig 8.6b (above): Right rotation of the SBS about an AP axis.

NOTE: the above strains (RT, LT, SBR$_L$, SBR$_R$) are all considered physiologic if their presence does not interfere with the flexion or extension components of the mechanism. [1 p.906]

Copyright 1999

C. Flexion/Extension

As mentioned earlier, flexion and extension are natural physiologic components of the C.R.I. A strain pattern occurs when the mechanism does not move through flexion and extension equally., *An extension lesion occurs when the SBS deviates caudad, decreasing the amount of flexion of the C.R.I.* (Fig 8.7a). *Conversely, a flexion lesion occurs when the SBS is deviates cephalad, decreasing the amount of extension of the C.R.I* (Fig 8.7b).

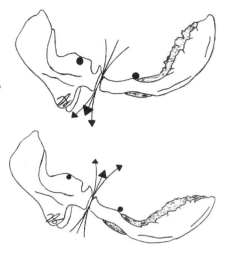

Fig 8.7a (above right): Extension of the SBS: The SBS deviates caudad (arrows) decreasing the amount of flexion in the C.R.I.
Fig 8.7b (right): Flexion of the SBS: The SBS deviates cephalad (arrows) decreasing the amount of extension in the C.R.I.

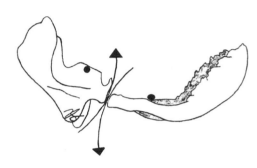

D. Vertical strain

A vertical strain of the SBS is present when the sphenoid deviates cephalad (superior vertical strain) or caudad (inferior vertical strain) in relation to the occiput. Rotation will occur about two transverse axes. One through the center of the sphenoid, the other superior to the occiput. Rotation of the sphenoid and the occiput about these axes are in the same direction.

Fig 8.8: Superior vertical strain: The sphenoid deviates cephalad in relation to the occiput.

E. Lateral strain

A lateral strain of the SBS is present when the sphenoid deviates laterally in relation to the occiput. If the sphenoid deviates to the left, it is termed a left lateral strain. If the sphenoid deviates to the right, it is termed a right lateral strain. Rotation will occur about two vertical axes, one through the center of the sphenoid, the other through foramen magnum. Rotation of the sphenoid and the occiput about these axes are in the same direction. Palpation of a lateral strain will feel as if the cranium is shaped like a parallelogram.

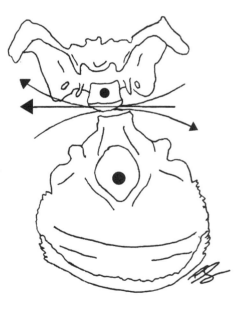

Fig 8.9: Left lateral strain: The sphenoid deviates laterally in relation to the occiput.

NOTE: Vertical and lateral strains may be superimposed on other strains.

F. Compression

SBS compression is present when the sphenoid and the occiput have been forced together (usually due to trauma to the back of the head). *This type of strain prevents physiologic flexion and extension. Therefore, the C.R.I. is absent upon palpation.*

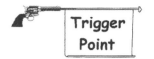

> **Compression strain of the SBS will result in no C.R.I. It is usually due to trauma, especially to the back of the head.**

IV. Cranial nerves

Table 8.1 Summary of the cranial nerves

Nerve	Exits the Cranium through the	Somatic dysfunction	Symptoms associated with Somatic Dysfunction.
CN I	Cribiform plate	Sphenoid, frontal, ethmoid	Altered sense of smell
CN II	Otic canal	Sphenoid, occiput	Visual changes
CN III	Superior orbital fissure	Sphenoid, temporal	Diplopia, ptosis or accommodation problems
CN IV	Superior orbital fissure	Sphenoid, temporal	Diplopia when looking down
CN V V_1	Superior orbital fissure	Sphenoid, temporal	Dec. sensation to upper eyelid and scalp
V_2	Foramen rotundum	Sphenoid, temporal, maxillae, mandible	Symptoms similar to Tic Douloureux
V_3	Foramen ovale	Sphenoid	Dec. sensation to mandible and tenderpoints within the muscles of mastication
CN VI	Superior orbital fissure	Sphenoid, temporal	Diplopia
CN VII	Enters the internal acoustic meatus and exits the stylomastoid foramen	Sphenoid, temporal, occiput	Symptoms similar to Bell's palsy
CN VIII	Internal acoustic meatus	Sphenoid, temporal, occiput	Tinnitus, vertigo or hearing loss
CN IX	Jugular foramen	Temporal, occiput	
CN X	Jugular foramen	Temporal, occiput, OA, AA, C2	Headaches, arrhythmias, GI upset, respiratory problems
CN XI	Spinal division (C1-C6) enters foramen magnum joins with the cranial division and exits the jugular foramen	Temporal, occiput	Tenderness in the SCM or trapezius
CN XII	Hypoglossal canal	Occiput	Dysphagia

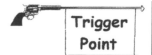

> 1. **Vagal somatic dysfunction can be due to OA, AA and/or C2 dysfunction.**
> 2. **Dysfunction of CN VIII can cause tinnitus, vertigo or hearing loss.**

V. Craniosacral treatment

The goal of craniosacral treatment is to reduce venous congestion, mobilize articular restrictions, balance the SBS and enhance the rate and amplitude of the C.R.I. [14 p.171] Although treatment varies from practitioner to practitioner, there are some general techniques that every osteopathic physician should be familiar with in order to treat the patient successfully. All of the following techniques ultimately depend upon the inherent motility of the brain and spinal cord to reestablish normal mobility. For a full description of the craniosacral techniques see Greenman's Principles of Manual Medicine Chapter 12 pages 169-170.

A. Venous sinus technique

Purpose - To increase venous flow through the venous sinuses so that blood may exit the skull through the jugular foramen. [14 p.169]

B. CV4: Bulb decompression

Purpose - To enhance the amplitude of the C.R.I., by first resisting the flexion and extension of the occiput until a "still point" is reached, then allowing restoration of normal flexion and extension. [14 p.169-70]

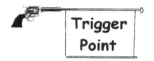

Trigger Point

> **The CV4 will increase the amplitude of the C.R.I.**

C. Vault hold

Purpose - To address the strains at the SBS. The operator can use either a direct or indirect method of treatment. Most commonly, an indirect method is used to balance membranous tension. [14 p.170]

D. V spread

Purpose - To separate restricted or impacted sutures. The principle can be applied to any suture. [14 p.170]

E. Lift technique

Purpose - Frontal and parietal lifts are commonly used to aid in the balance of membranous tension. [14 p.170]

VI. Indications for craniosacral treatment

Craniosacral treatment can be used for common strain patterns caused by any stresses that disturb the PRM. Craniosacral treatment can also be used in the following scenarios:

1. After the birth of a child

    Trauma to the cranial bones often occurs during delivery. Craniosacral treatment within the first few days of life facilitates bony remodeling of the skull. If no treatment is given and sutures continue to overlap, the cranial bones will grow together, forming a synostosis. [1 p.909]

2. Trauma to the PRM

    This can occur from mild forces, such as orthodontics or severe forces such as a car accident. Regardless of the cause, the PRM will remain compromised. Craniosacral treatment should be directed at normalizing the rate and amplitude of the C.R.I.

3. Dentistry

    Extraction of teeth, the filling of cavities, or improperly fitted dentures can compromise the PRM. Headaches, vertigo or TMJ dysfunction may result from improperly directed forces associated with dentistry. [1 p.911]

A. <u>Complications</u>

Although uncommon, headaches, tinnitus, or dizziness has been reported following some treatments. SBS strain treatment may cause an alteration in heart rate, blood pressure, respiration, and gastrointestinal irritability. [14 p.171]

B. <u>Contraindications</u>

1. <u>Absolute contraindications</u>
   a. Acute intracranial bleed or increased intracranial pressure
   b. Skull fracture

2. <u>Relative contraindications</u>
   a. In patients with known seizure history or dystonia, great care must be used in order not exacerbate any neurological symptoms.
   b. Traumatic brain injury

Chapter 9
Facilitation

I. Facilitation

Definition - the maintenance of a pool of neurons (e.g., premotor neurons, motoneurons of preganglionic sympathetic neurons in one or more segments of the spinal cord) in a state of partial or sub-threshold excitation. In this state, less afferent stimulation is required to trigger the discharge of impulses. Facilitation may be due to a sustained increase in afferent input, or changes within the affected neurons themselves, or their chemical environment. Once established, facilitation can be sustained by normal CNS activity. [1 p.1130]

A. Neurophysiologic mechanism of facilitation

If facilitation occurs at an individual spinal level it is termed segmental facilitation. In order to closely examine segmental facilitation we must first look at the spinal reflex. A spinal reflex is thought to have three simple parts: [15 p.65]

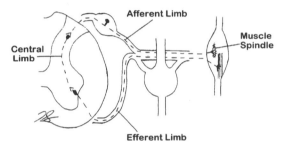

1. An afferent limb (sensory input)
2. A central limb (spinal pathway)
3. An efferent limb (motor pathway)

Fig 9.1: Simplification of a spinal reflex: Sensory input is transmitted by a afferent limb, processed by the central limb (interneurons) then a motor response is transmitted by the efferent limb.

Unfortunately, this is an oversimplification. In actuality, sensory input originates from many places causing a variety of effects throughout the spinal cord. Within the spinal cord, ascending/descending, branching, and crossing interneurons process (and further complicate) the sensory information. Output at the spinal segment could be to lower motor neurons (dorsal/ventral rami) to muscle or to viscera via the autonomic nervous system. Thus, a spinal reflex is actually part of a vast ever-changing network of neurons that is finely tuned to regulate the activity of the body. [15 p.65]

B. How does a segment become (and stay) facilitated? (Figs 9.2 a,b)

A spinal cord segment can receive input from three areas:
1. From higher centers (brain).
2. From viscera via sympathetic or parasympathetic visceral afferents.
3. From somatic afferents (muscle spindles, golgi tendons, nociceptors, etc.).

Any abnormal and steady sensory stimulus from one of these three areas can cause the interneurons at a spinal cord level to become sensitive to the stimulus. These "sensitized" interneurons will have an increased or exaggerated output to the initiating site as well as other areas (neighboring muscles, or organs via autonomic efferents). Once the sensitized state is established, the segment is then considered to be facilitated. Any continuous sensitizing input or the presence of normal input through sensitized interneurons, will maintain the process allowing the abnormal situation to continue.

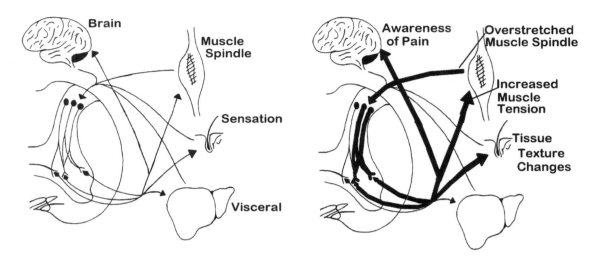

Fig 9.2a (above left): Normal afferent and efferent circuit . Fig 9.2b (above right): Facilitated segment: An abnormal sensory stimulus from an overstretched muscle spindle sensitizes two interneurons in the spinal cord. This will result in an increased or exaggerated output to the initiating site (resulting in increased muscle tension), as well as the brain (resulting in an awareness of pain), and local cutaneous tissue (resulting in tissue texture changes).

C. How does facilitation correlate with somatic dysfunction?

Let us investigate what might occur when a patient strains his deltoid muscle.

1. Abnormal and continuous sensory input from the overstretched muscle spindle sensitizes the interneurons in the spinal cord at C5.

2. A reflex occurs so that muscle tension is produced at the deltoid muscle. This will result in a **restricted** range of motion of the deltoid and **tenderness** upon palpation.

3. Prolonged muscle tension causes continuation of the sensitizing input, and the maintenance of the facilitated segment.

4. Muscle tension at the initiation site (deltoid) causes nociceptor activation in the neighboring areas, and a release of bradykinins, serotonin, histamines, potassium, prostaglandins, substance P, and leukotrienes. [1 p.917] These substances will cause local vasodilatation and **tissue texture changes.**

5. The abnormal and continuous sensory input into C5 may also cause a paraspinal muscle spasm. The facilitated interneurons may cause an exaggerated motor output through the dorsal rami at C5 causing increased muscle tension in the deep paraspinal muscles. The resulting increase in muscle tension will cause C5, to rotate or sidebend so that **asymmetry** is present.

6. Therefore, a facilitated segment can lead to:

> 1. **T**enderness.
>
> 2. **A**symmetry.
>
> 3. **R**estriction.
>
> 4. **T**issue texture change.

TART = the diagnostic criteria for somatic dysfunction.

D. Reflexes

1. **Viscero-somatic reflex** (Fig 9.3)

According to the Glossary of Osteopathic Terminology, a viscero-somatic reflex occurs when localized visceral stimuli produce patterns of reflex response, in segmentally related somatic structures. For example, acute cholecystitis often refers pain to the mid-thoracic region at the tip of the right scapula.

2. **Somato-visceral reflex**

Somatic stimuli may produce patterns of reflex response in segmentally related visceral structures. For example, a tenderpoint located in the right pectoralis major muscle, between the fifth and sixth ribs and just medial to the nipple line, has been known to cause supraventricular tachyarrhythmias. [1] p.931

Although viscero-somatic and somato-visceral reflexes are probably the most common, other reflexes are also possible. They include: somato-somatic, viscero-visceral, psycho-somatic, and psycho-visceral reflexes.

E. How does facilitation correlate with these reflexes?

Lets investigate how acute cholecystitis can cause referred pain to the mid-thoracic region at the tip of the right scapula, and somatic dysfunction of T5- T9 (a common viscero-somatic reflex).

1. Continued gallbladder dysfunction, most often caused by gallstones, [8] p.926 will transmit an abnormal sensory input (from visceral receptors) into the spinal cord. This will result in segmental facilitation of T5- T9.

2. Normal sensory input from general afferents (e.g., muscle spindle) at T5- T9 will become amplified at the sensitized interneurons, resulting in an exaggerated motor response. This will cause an increase in tension in the paraspinal musculature of T5 - T9. Tenderness and pain can then be elicited at this region.

3. In addition, the increased muscle tension in the paraspinal muscles, will cause T5 - T9 to rotate and sidebend so that somatic dysfunction is present.

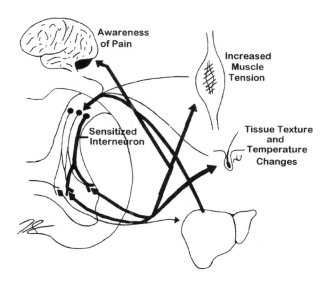

Fig 9.3: Viscero-somatic reflex: Continued visceral dysfunction will transmit abnormal sensory input into the spinal cord, resulting in facilitation of the interneurons. This will result in an exaggerated efferent response to somatic structures and the brain.

NOTE: Another common viscero-somatic reflex is T1-T5 somatic dysfunction, and pain radiating into the jaw and left arm, associated with cardiac dysfunction.

II. **Autonomic innervation**

Since visceral dysfunction transmits information to the spinal cord via autonomic afferents, it is essential for the osteopathic physician to understand the somatic areas likely to show effects of underlying visceral pathologic conditions through viscero-somatic reflexes. [1 p.572] Table 9.1 demonstrates the effects of the autonomic nervous system on various organ systems. Fig 9.4 on the following page details the visceral innervation of the parasympathetic nervous system. Table 9.2 shows the visceral innervation of the sympathetic nervous system.

Table 9.1 [13 p.275, 16 p.250, 17 p.672]

Structure	Parasympathetic Function	Sympathetic Function
Eye		
Pupil	Constricts (miosis)	Dilates (mydriasis)
Lens	Contracts for near vision	Slight relaxation for far vision
Glands		
Nasal, lacrimal, parotid, submandibular, gastric and pancreatic	Stimulates copious secretion (containing many enzymes for enzyme secreting glands)	Vasoconstriction for slight secretion
Sweat glands	Sweating on palms of hands	Copious sweating (cholinergic)
Heart	Decreases contractility and conduction velocity	Increases contractility and conduction velocity
Lungs		
Bronchiolar smooth muscle	Contracts	Relaxes
GI tract		
Smooth muscle		
Lumen	Contracts	Relaxes
Sphincters	Relaxes	Contracts
Secretion and motility	Increases	Decreases
Systemic arterioles		
Skin and visceral vessels	None	Contracts
Skeletal muscle	None	Relaxes
Genitourinary		
Bladder wall (detrusor)	Contracts	
Bladder sphincter (trigone)	Relaxes	Contracts
Penis	Erection	Ejaculation
Adrenal medulla		Secretes catacholamines
Liver		Gluconeogenesis and Glycogenolysis

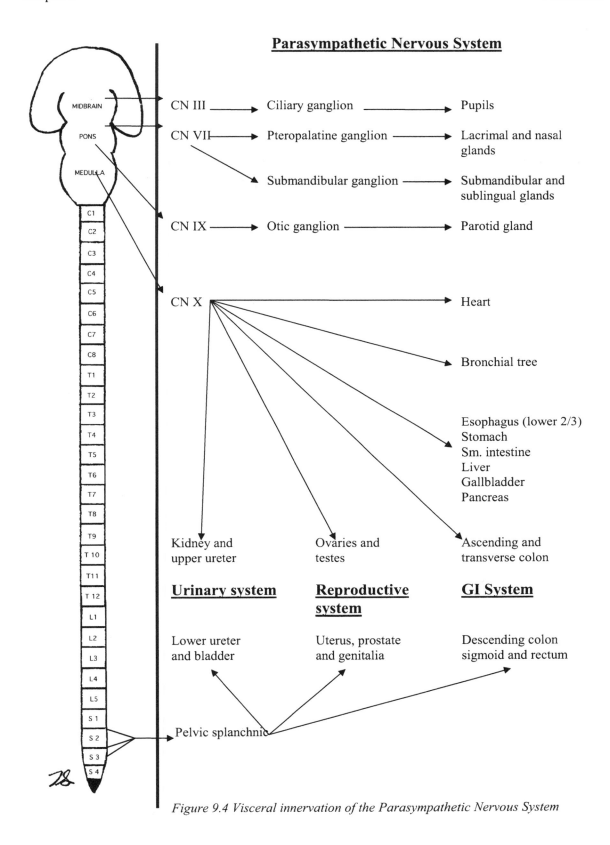

Figure 9.4 Visceral innervation of the Parasympathetic Nervous System

Sympathetic Nervous System

NOTE: Segmental sympathetic innervation varies from individual to individual and consequently will vary from author to author. There is no need to memorize the exact innervation for all the organs, but rather become familiar with the region of the spinal cord that innervates the viscera.

Table 9.2 [1 p.56, 18 p.459]

Visceral Organ	Spinal Cord Level	Corresponding Nerve (if any)	Corresponding Ganglion (if any)
Head and neck	T1 - T4		
Heart	T1 - T5		
Respiratory system	T2 - T7		
Esophagus	T2 - T8		

Upper GI tract
    Stomach
    Liver
    Gallbladder
    Spleen
    Portions of the pancreas
      and duodenum
	T5 - T9	Greater splanchnic nerve	Ciliac ganglion

Middle GI tract
    Portions of the pancreas
      and duodenum
    Jejunum
    Ilium
    Ascending colon
    Proximal 2/3 of
      transverse colon
	T9 - T12	Lesser splanchnic nerve	Superior mesenteric ganglion

Lower GI tract
    Distal 1/3 of transverse
      colon
    Descending colon
    Sigmoid colon
    Rectum
	T12 - L2	Least splanchnic nerve	Inferior mesenteric

Kidneys	T11 - L1		
Adrenal medulla	T10		
Upper ureters	T10 - L1		
Lower ureters	L1 - L2		
Bladder	T11 - L2		
Gonads	T10 - T11		
Uterus and cervix	T10 - L2		
Erectile tissue of penis and clitoris	T11 - L2		

Extremities
    Arms
    Legs
	
	T5 - T7[1 p.61]
	T10 - L2		

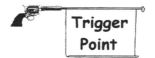

| Trigger Point | It is essential for anyone taking the COMLEX boards to understand the segmental innervation to each visceral organ. Approximately 20% of the boards questions will stem from Fig 9.4 and Table 9.2. |

A. Key points concerning autonomic innervations

1. **Parasympathetic**

   a. The vagus nerve innervates:
   - ◊ The entire thoracic region.
   - ◊ The abdominal region up to the proximal half of the transverse colon.
   - ◊ Only the kidneys, upper 1/2 of the ureters, and testes or ovaries in the pelvic region.

   b. The pelvic splanchnic nerves innervate:
   - ◊ The distal half of the transverse colon to the rectum.
   - ◊ All of the pelvic organs except the small portion that the vagus innervates.

   NOTE: The adrenals and extremities have no parasympathetic innervation.

2. **Sympathetic**

   a. T1-T4:
   - ◊ Head and neck

   b. T1-T5:
   - ◊ Heart

   c. T2 - T7:
   - ◊ Lungs

   d. T5-L2:
   - ◊ Entire GI tract

   e. T5-T7:
   - ◊ Upper Extremities

NOTE: T9-T12 = the superior mesenteric ganglion. This innervates a portion of the pancreas, to the proximal half of the transverse colon. Anything above this is T5-T9, anything below T12-L2.

   f. L3-L5:
   - ◊ **NOTHING**!! (The spinal cord only extends to L2 in a normal adult)

Chapter 10
Chapman's Reflexes and Travell's Myofascial Trigger points

I. Chapman's Reflexes

Chapman's reflexes are a system of reflex points originated by Frank Chapman, D.O. These reflexes are predictable tissue texture abnormalities assumed to be a reflection of visceral dysfunction or pathology. [1 p.1128]

Starting in the 1920's, Frank Chapman D.O. discovered that specific "ganglioform contractions" were associated with visceral dysfunction. [19] These "ganglioform contractions" which were later called Chapman's reflex points, are *smooth, firm, discretely palpable nodules, approximately 2-3 mm in diameter located within the deep fascia or on the periostium of a bone.* When a Chapman reflex point is located by the examiner, gentle pressure will usually elicit a sharp, nonradiating, and exquisitely distressing pain. [1 p.936]

Chapman's reflexes, in current clinical practice, are used more for diagnosis than for treatment. *They are thought to represent viscero-somatic reflexes.* Palpating for a Chapman's reflex point can often provide the physician with clinical evidence of the presence or absence of visceral disease.

A. Important Chapman's reflex points

Table 10.1

Reflex point	Location
1. **Appendix**	**At the tip of the right 12th rib.** **The presence of this particular reflex point helps to direct the differential diagnosis more toward acute appendicitis.
2. Adrenals	2" superior and 1" lateral to the umbilicus and/or the spinous process of T11.
3. Kidneys	1" superior and 1" lateral to the umbilicus and/or the spinous process of L1.
4. Bladder	At the umbilicus.
5. Colon	Along the femur.

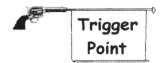

Trigger Point

The appendix Chapman's point is located at the tip of the 12th rib.

II. Travell's Myofascial Trigger Points

A trigger point is a hypersensitive focus, usually within a taut band of skeletal muscle or in the muscle fascia. It is painful upon compression and can give rise to a characteristic referred pain, tenderness, and autonomic phenomena. [20 p. 3]

A. Diagnostic characteristics

The patient may complain of tightness or soreness in a particular muscle that may or may not have followed an injury. On examination, the physician can palpate a taut band within the muscle. Upon compression of the band, the patient will experience pain at the site *and pain referring to an area of the body*. This referred pain is reproducible and specific for certain muscles. For example, trigger points located within the sternocleidomastoid will refer pain to occipital and temporal regions ipsilaterally. [20]

B. Pathophysiology

The spinal cord plays an important role in the establishment and maintenance of trigger points. Direct stimuli, such as a muscular strain, overwork fatigue, or postural imbalance, can initiate trigger points. [1 p.916] This concept is very similar to facilitation. For example, if a person were to strain his deltoid, abnormal and continuous sensory input from the overstretched muscle spindle will sensitize the interneurons at C5. A reflex occurs so that muscle tension is produced within the deltoid at the initiating site, resulting in a taut band. If this taut band refers pain when compressed, then it is considered a trigger point. Other stimuli, such as visceral dysfunction, may also facilitate the spinal cord. Sixty-one percent of patients with cardiac disease were reported to have chest muscle trigger points. [20 p.586] Conversely, trigger points may facilitate the spinal cord and cause visceral dysfunction. [1 p.917]

C. Treatment

Myofascial trigger points can be treated in many ways. All techniques are directed toward eliminating the trigger point using a neurological or vascular method. The following procedures have been successful in eliminating trigger points: [21 p.9-10]

- ◊ Spray and stretch using vapocoolant spray
- ◊ Injection with local anesthetic or dry needling
- ◊ Muscle energy techniques
- ◊ Myofascial release
- ◊ Ultrasound
- ◊ High voltage galvanic stimulation
- ◊ Reciprocal inhibition
- ◊ Ischemic compression

D. Trigger point vs. tenderpoint

Tenderpoints were first introduced by Lawerence Jones, D.O. Tenderpoints are small, hypersensitive points in the myofascial tissues of the body used as diagnostic criteria, and as a treatment monitor for counterstrain (Glossary of Osteopathic Terminology). Tenderpoints are similar to trigger points in that they are taut myofascial bands that are painful upon compression. *However, tenderpoints do not refer pain beyond the location compressed.* Some authors note a significant overlap in the location between trigger points and tenderpoints, [22] while some authors state that their distinction is somewhat arbitrary. [23]

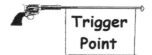

Trigger points refer pain when pressed.
Tenderpoints DO NOT refer pain when pressed.

Chapter **11**
Myofascial Release

I. <u>Myofascial Release</u>

Myofascial Release is a form of manual medicine that combines several types of OMT in order to stretch and release muscle (myo) and fascia (fascial) restrictions. Counterstrain, facilitated positional release, unwinding, balanced ligamentous release, functional indirect release, direct fascial release, cranial osteopathy, and visceral manipulation are all forms of myofascial release. [25 p.380] Since counterstrain and facilitated positional release have unique features, they are discussed separately in the next chapter.

Myofascial release treatment can be direct or indirect, active or passive (see chapter 1 The Basics for a further explanation of these types of treatment). It also can be performed anywhere from head to toe, because fascia surrounds and compartmentalizes all structures throughout the body. For this reason, there are several hundred different types of myofascial release techniques. It is not in the scope of this text to describe all of these treatments, but rather, a typical myofascial release procedure will be outlined, along with two very common myofascial release techniques.

A. <u>Typical Myofascial Release Treatment</u>
1. The physician must first palpate a restriction.
   A restriction may present itself as muscle tension, tenderness or decreased movement of an articulation.

2. Once a restriction is palpated, the physician must then decide the type of treatment.
   In a direct treatment, the physician will move myofascial tissues toward a restrictive barrier. This can be accomplished by using a limb as a lever and monitoring tissue tension at the restriction, or it can be accomplished by directly applying a **traction** along the long axis of the muscle.
   In an indirect treatment, the physician will move myofascial structures away from the restrictive barrier. Again, this can be accomplished by using a limb as a lever, or by applying a **compression** along the long axis of the muscle.

3. Then the physician will add other forces to "fine tune" the treatment.
   Twisting the myofascial structures (clockwise or counter-clockwise)or applying **transverse forces** perpendicular to the long axis of the muscle are added in a direct or indirect fashion. Also, passive movement of a limb may aid in the fine tuning of the myofascial treatment.

4. After the physician has correctly addressed the myofascial structures, the patient is asked to use "enhancers" to help induce a release.
   Enhancers include active movement of the patient (respiration, eye movement or muscle contraction). Again, these movements are added in a direct or indirect fashion.

5. The physician then awaits a release. A release may come in many forms, a change in temperature, a tightness may "melt" or "give way". The release may occur at different levels of the fascia or in several directions. The release phenomena is subtle and can only be appreciated by the skilled practitioner. Therefore, it may take several attempts before the osteopathic student can experience the release phenomenon.

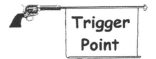

> ## Myofascial release procedure
> 1. **Palpate restriction**
> 2. **Apply compression (indirect) or traction (direct)**
> 3. **Add twisting or transverse forces**
> 4. **Use enhancers**
> 5. **Await release**

B. Goal of Myofascial Release
1) Restore functional balance to all integrative tissues in the musculoskeletal system.
2) **Improve lymphatic flow** by removing myofascial restrictions.

C. Indications and Contraindications

Indications - Myofascial release techniques are typically gentle and can be performed on acutely ill hospitalized patients and elderly patients who cannot tolerate more aggressive therapy. Since these techniques can be done in multiple positions, they also can be done on those patients who cannot tolerate much movement.

Since myofascial release will improve lymphatic return, it can be beneficial in the following conditions:
1. CHF
2. Asthma
3. COPD

Relative Contraindications [1 p.947]
1. Bacterial infection (especially if temp $> 102^0$)
2. Osseous fracture
3. Advanced stages of cancer (risk of spread of metastatic disease)
4. Traumatic disruption of visceral organs

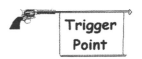

> Lymphatic techniques (pedal pump, thoracic pump, etc.) as well as some myofascial release techniques are contraindicated in patients with cancer due to an increased risk of lymphogenous spread. [1 p.428]

D. Physiologic diaphragms
There are four diaphragms in the human body. All play a role in lymphatic return (the most important being the abdominal diaphragm).

The four diaphragms are:

Tentorium cerebelli

Thoracic inlet

Abdominal diaphragm

Pelvic diaphragm

E. Diaphragm Release Techniques

Thoracic Inlet Release (a.k.a. thoracic outlet release)
Purpose - To relax soft tissue restrictions and enhance lymphatic drainage from the head and neck.

Procedure:
Direct myofascial release procedure. [1 p.949]
1. Patient supine with arm abducted to 90^0.
2. Physician seated at the side of the patient.
3. With one hand, place your fingers in the patient's supraclavicular fossa and apply traction towards the patient's wrist.
4. With the other hand, move the patient's wrist superiorly until tension develops in the supraclavicular fossa. Hold this until some relaxation is noted.
5. Repeat this procedure two to three times.

Thoracoabdominal Diaphragm Release
Purpose - To increase pressure gradients within the thoracic and abdominal cavities, thereby increasing lymphatic return. [1 p.951] There are several different types of thoracoabdominal release, the following is example of an indirect myofascial release.

Procedure:
1. Patient seated
2. Physician standing behind patient.
3. Pass your hands around the thoracic cage (under the patient's arms) and introduce your fingers underneath the costal margin.
4. Test for motion by gently rotating the thoracic tissues.
5. Treatment phase: With your fingers still underneath the costal margin, hold the thoracic tissues in the direction which it moves more freely. Allow the fascia to unwind, until it settles into a rhythmic vertical motion.

II. Fascial Patterns (Common Compensatory Patterns)

Many authors have noted that the musculoskeletal system in most individuals is asymmetric. These authors postulate that fascias of the body have a tendency to rotate in a certain direction. The fascia at one area will rotate one way, and the fascia in another area will rotate the opposite direction to compensate. J.Gordon Zink, D.O. was the first to provide documented material about these fascial preferences. Zink states that there are four compensatory curves throughout the spine. [1 p.946]

They are:
1. Occipitoatlantal junction
2. Cervicothoracic junction
3. Thoracolumbar junction
4. Lumbosacral junction

Rotatory testing of these segments reveal that in approximately 80% of **healthy individuals** the OA is rotated left, the cervicothoracic rotated right, the thoracolumbar rotated left and the lumbosacral rotated right. *Zink called this the Common Compensatory Pattern.* The remainder of **healthy individuals** (20%) had the opposite pattern. *Zink called this the Uncommon Compensatory Pattern.* He also noticed that unhealthy individuals, such as hospitalized patients, or those patients that recently experienced a traumatic event or stress, did not show this type of alternating pattern. In other words, their fascial preference did not alternate in direction from one reference area to the next. [28 p.46]

Table 11.1

Junction	Common Compensatory Pattern (80%) Rotation	Uncommon Compensatory Pattern (20%) Rotation
Occipitoatlantal	Left	Right
Cervicothoracic	Right	Left
Thoracolumbar	Left	Right
Lumbosacral	Right	Left

Chapter 12

Counterstrain and Facilitated Positional Release (FPR)

Counterstrain

I. Definition

   *Counterstrain is a **passive indirect technique** in which the tissue being treated is positioned at a point of balance, or ease, away from the restrictive barrier.* [1 p. 809] Counterstrain was pioneered by Lawerence H. Jones in 1955. Jones discovered that by placing a patient in a position of ease for 90 seconds he could eliminate "tenderpoints." He initially referred to this new treatment approach as "spontaneous release by positioning". He later called it strain counterstrain, or simply counterstrain. [1 p.810]

A. What is a tenderpoint?
   A tenderpoint is a small tense edematous area of tenderness about the size of a fingertip. [1 p. 811] They are typically located near bony attachments of tendons, ligaments or in the belly of some muscles. A trigger point is also a small, tense, hypersensitive area of tenderness. *However, trigger points will radiate pain to a specific area when compressed. Tenderpoints do not radiate pain to other locations of the body.*

B. Basic counterstrain treatment steps

   1. Locate a significant tenderpoint
      ◊ Tenderpoints can usually be found at the region of the patient's chief complaint. In addition, tenderpoints may also be located in a corresponding anterior location.
      ◊ Also keep in mind that pain at one location may be induced from a primary strain elsewhere. A common example of this is a patient with a psoas spasm complaining of low back pain. Although tenderness can be elicited at the lumbar spine and sacroiliac regions, a psoas tenderpoint located medial to the ASIS or periumbilical region will be present, and may be the cause of the lumbosacral pain.

   2. Palpate the tenderpoints.
      ◊ The pressure used to elicit a tenderpoint is only a few ounces.
      ◊ To determine if that point is clinically significant, compare the same spot to the other side.
      ◊ If there are multiple areas of tenderness, treat the most tender area first.

3. Place the patient in the position of optimal comfort.
   ◊ Maintaining light contact with the tenderpoint, the physician makes a gross adjustment **shortening the muscle** being treated.
   ◊ Reapply firm pressure to check for reduction of tenderness.
   ◊ Fine tune the treatment with small areas of motion until at least 70% of the tenderness has been reduced.

   ### Maverick Point
   Approximately 5% of tenderpoints will not improve with the expected treatment even with careful fine tuning. These Maverick points are treated by positioning the patient a position opposite of what would be used typically. [1 p.812]

4. With the patient completely relaxed, maintain the position of comfort for 90 seconds.
   ◊ Ninety seconds is the time required for the proprioceptive firing to decrease in frequency and amplitude. [25 p.88-9]

5. Slow return to neutral.
   ◊ The first few degrees are the most important. [1 p. 813]
   ◊ Make sure the patient is completely relaxed and does not try to help by actively moving.

6. Recheck the tenderpoint.
   ◊ No more than 30% of the tenderness should remain.
   ◊ Tenderness from a viscerosomatic reflex will return within a few hours. [1 p.813]

II. Counterstrain techniques
A. Cervical Spine

Anterior Cervical Tenderpoints
Location:
The lateral aspect or slightly anterior to the lateral mass (articular pillar) of the vertebrae [1 p.815]

Treatment position:
Sidebend and rotate the patient's head away from the side of the tenderpoint.

Posterior Cervical Tenderpoints
Location:
Usually at the tip of the spinous process or on the lateral sides of the spinous process.

Treatment Position:
Extend, sidebend (slightly), and rotate away.

NOTE: The cervical spine has the greatest number of maverick tenderpoints.

B. Thoracic Spine

Anterior Thoracic Tenderpoints
Location:
T1-T6: Located at the midline of the sternum at the attachment of the corresponding ribs
T7-T12: Most are located in the rectus abdominus muscle about one inch lateral to the midline on the right or left.

Treatment Position:
Flex thorax and add a small amount of sidebending and rotation away.

Posterior Thoracic Tenderpoints
> Location:
> > On either side of the spinous process or on the transverse process.

> Treatment Position
> > Extend, rotate away and sidebend slightly away.

C. Ribs

Anterior tenderpoints are associated with anteriorly depressed ribs (also called exhalation ribs, an exhalation dysfunction, or an inhalation restriction). Posterior tenderpoints are associated with posteriorly depressed ribs (also called inhalation ribs, an inhalation dysfunction, or an exhalation restriction) [1 p.815]

Anterior Rib Tenderpoints
> Location:
> > Rib 1: Tenderpoint is located just below the medial end of the clavicle.
> > Rib 2: Tenderpoint is 6-8cm lateral to the sternum on rib 2 [26 p.78]

> > Ribs 3-6: Are located along the mid-axillary line on the corresponding rib.

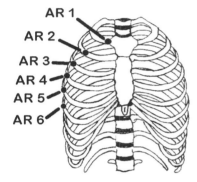

> Treatment Position:
> > Rib 1 and 2: Flex head, sidebend and rotate towards.
> > Ribs 3-6: Sidebend and rotate the thorax toward, encourage slight flexion.

Posterior Rib Tenderpoints

Fig 12.1: Anterior rib tenderpoints

> Location:
> > The angle of the corresponding rib.

> Treatment Position:
> > Most of these are treated with minimal flexion, sidebend away and rotation away. Jones recommends maintaining rib treatment positions for 120 seconds to allow the patient extra time to relax. [1 p.815]

D. Lumbar Spine
Anterior Lumbar Tenderpoints
> Location:
> > L1: Medial to the ASIS.
> > L2-L4: On the AIIS.
> > L5: One cm lateral to the pubic symphysis on the superior ramus.

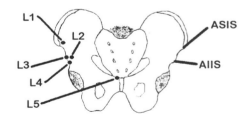

Fig 12.2: Anterior lumbar tenderpoints

> Treatment Position:
> > Most are treated with the patient supine, knees and hips flexed and markedly rotated away .

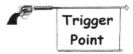

The anterior tenderpoint for L5 is located one cm lateral to the pubic symphysis on the superior ramus.

Posterior Lumbar Tenderpoints

Location:

On either side of the spinous process or on the transverse process. L3 and L4 may be found on the iliac crest. Also, L5 may be found on the PSIS.

Treatment Position:

Most are treated with the patient prone, extended and sidebent away (rotation may be towards or away).

E. Pelvis

There are many tenderpoints for pelvic muscles and associated structures. Perhaps the most important of these is the iliacus.

Iliacus:

Location:

Approximately 7 cm medial to the ASIS.

Treatment Position:

Patient supine with the hip flexed and externally rotated.

Facilitated Positional Release (FPR)

A. Definition

A system of indirect myofascial release treatment developed by Stanley Schiowitz, D.O. The component region of the body is placed into a neutral position, diminishing tissue and joint tension, in all planes, and an activating force (compression or torsion) is added. [1 p.1133] It is easily applied, nontraumatic and only takes 3-4 seconds to induce a release.

FPR Technique can be used to treat:

1. Superficial muscles
2. Deep intervertebral muscles to influence vertebral motion

Typical FPR Procedure

Superficial Muscle Treatment

1. With the patient in a relaxed position, the physician first straightens the AP curvature of the spine (decreasing the kyphosis or lordosis).
2. The physician then applies the facilitating force (compression or torsion, or both).
3. The physician then shortens the muscle to be treated.
4. The position is held for 3 to 4 seconds.
5. The physician releases the position and reevaluates the dysfunction.

Deep intervertebral muscle treatment (Intervertebral motion treatment)

Diagnosis C5 ES_RR_R:

1. The patient is supine, with his/her head beyond the end of the table, resting in a pillow in the physician's lap.
2. With the patient in a relaxed position, straighten the cervical lordosis by flexing the head slightly.
3. The physician then applies the facilitating force (compression or torsion, or both).
4. The physician will then place C5 in ES_RR_R using the head as a lever.
5. The position is held for 3 to 4 seconds.
6. The physician releases the position and reevaluates the dysfunction.

Chapter 13
Muscle Energy

Daniel G. Bersen

I. Definition
A form of OMT in which the patient actively uses his muscles, on request, "from a precisely controlled position in a specific direction, against a distinctly executed counterforce." [1 p.1133]

II. Principles of Muscle Energy Treatment
Muscle energy can be performed as an **active direct** or **active indirect** techniques (see chapter 1 The Basics for further description of these types of treatments).

NOTE: Most forms of muscle energy treatment are direct. Indirect is rarely used.

*The **direct technique** utilizes **postisometric relaxation** to correct somatic dysfunction.*
*The **indirect technique** utilizes **reciprocal inhibition** to correct somatic dysfunction.*

III. Types of Muscle Energy

1. Postisometric relaxation (direct technique): The physician, after correct diagnosis of the somatic dysfunction, reverses all components in all planes and engages the restrictive barrier.
   ◊ The physician then instructs the patient to contract equally against the offered counterforce by the physician. This isometric contraction where the distance between the origin and the insertion of the muscle remains the same as the muscle contracts will stretch the internal connective tissues.
   ◊ The golgi tendon organs senses this change in tension in the muscle tendons and causes a reflex relaxation of the agonist muscle fibers. [1 p.694] Therefore, by reflex relaxation of the agonist muscle, the physician is then able to passively stretch the patient in all planes of motion to the new restrictive barrier.
   ◊ For example, if the biceps muscle is in spasm, extend the elbow fully to the restrictive barrier, flex the biceps against resistance for 3-5 seconds, then relax. Extend the elbow to the new restrictive barrier then repeat.

2. Reciprocal inhibition (indirect technique): Another muscle energy technique utilizes the reflex mechanism of reciprocal inhibition when antagonistic muscles are contracted.
   ◊ By contracting the antagonistic muscle, signals are transmitted to the spinal cord and through the reciprocal inhibition reflex arc, the agonist muscle is then forced to relax.
   ◊ For example, if the biceps muscle is in spasm, have the patient flex the antagonistic muscle, the triceps, against resistance. This isometric force through reciprocal inhibition allows the biceps muscle to relax and return to a normal resting state.

IV. <u>Muscle Energy Treatment Procedure</u>

1. The physician positions the bone or joint so the muscle group will engage the restrictive barrier (direct treatment) in all planes of motion.
2. The operator instructs the patient to reverse direction in one or all planes of motion.
3. The patient contracts the appropriate muscle(s) or muscle group with the objective of moving the body part through a complete range of motion.
4. The physician maintains an appropriate counterforce so that the contraction is perceived at the **critical** articulation or area for 3-5 seconds.
5. The physician then instructs the patient to relax and the physician also relaxes. Then during the post-isometric relaxation phase, the physician takes up the slack, allowing it to be passively lengthened. Increased range of motion is noted by the physician.
6. Steps 1-5 are repeated for 3-5 times until the best possible increase in motion is obtained.

V. <u>Localization</u>

Localization of force is more important than intensity of force. Localization depends on the physician's palpatory perception of muscle activation (increased muscle tension) at a specific level. The physician must engage the restrictive barrier in all planes of motion. Such perception enables the operator to make subtle assessments about a dysfunction and to create variations of suggested treatment procedures.

VI. <u>Contraindications</u>

Muscle Energy should not be performed on patients with low vitality who could be further compromised by adding active muscular exertion. Examples of these types of patients are **post-surgical patients** and **intensive care patients.**[1 p.696]

VII. <u>Muscle Energy Techniques</u>

<u>Cervical Spine</u>

Positional Diagnosis: OA ES_LR_R
Treatment Position: Supine

1. With the distal pad of one finger monitor the OA joint, engage the restrictive barrier in all three planes by sidebending right, rotating left and flexing the patient's head until tension is felt under your monitoring finger. This is localization. Direct the patient to use a small amount of force to straighten his head while you exert an equal amount of counterforce.
2. Maintain the forces for 3-5 seconds, repeat 3-5 times, each time re-engaging the new restrictive barrier.
3. Recheck for symmetry of motion.

Positional Diagnosis: AA R_R
Treatment Position: Supine

1. Cradle the occiput in your hands and flex the patient's cervical spine 45^0, locking out all the facets below the AA joint.
2. Rotate the atlas to the left to the point of initial resistance.
3. Direct the patient to gently rotate their head to the right. Apply an equal counterforce through your fingers and hands.
4. Maintain the forces for 3-5 seconds, repeat 3-5 times, each time re-engaging the new restrictive barrier.
5. Recheck for symmetry of motion.

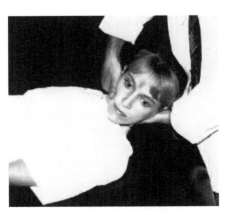

Fig 13.1: Treatment of AA R_R

Typical Cervicals (C2-C7)

1. With the distal pad of one finger on the articular pillar of the dysfunctional segment, engage the restrictive barrier by reversing the somatic dysfunction in all three planes of motion until motion is felt under your monitoring finger. Remember that *rotation and sidebending components are to the same side.*

2. Direct the patient to gently straighten their head while you apply an equal counterforce.

3. Repeat steps 4-5 in the above example.

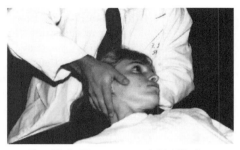

Fig 13.2: Treatment of C3 ER_RS_R

Thoracic Spine

Upper Thoracic Spine (T1-T4)
Positional Diagnosis: T3 ES_LR_L
Treatment Position: Seated

1. In the upper thoracic spine the physician will use the head as lever to induce motion at the dysfunctional segment.

2. With one hand monitor the posterior transverse process of T3. Engage the restrictive barrier by flexing, rotating and sidebending right until motion is felt under your monitoring finger.

3. Direct the patient to use a small amount of force to straighten their head while you exert an equal amount of counterforce.

4. Maintain the forces for 3-5 seconds, have the patient relax, the physician relaxes, and re-engage the new restrictive barrier.

5. Repeat step four 3-5 times and then recheck for increased symmetry.

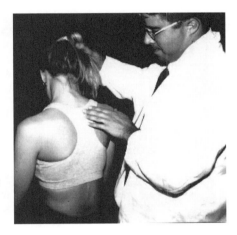

Fig 13.3: Treatment of T3 ES_LR_L

Lower Thoracic Spine (T5-T12)
Positional Diagnosis: T7 ER_LS_L
Treatment Position: Seated

1. Use your left hand to monitor the posterior transverse process of T7.

2. Instruct the patient to place their left hand behind their neck, and to grasp their left elbow with their right hand.

3. Reach across the patient's chest with your right arm, sidebending and rotating T7 to the right until motion is felt under your monitoring finger.

4. Direct the patient to use a small amount of force to straighten their body while you exert an equal amount of counterforce.

5. Repeat step four 3-5 times and then recheck for increased symmetry.

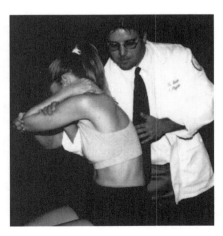

Fig 13.4: Treatment of T7 ER_LS_L

<u>Ribs</u>
Inhalation Dysfunctions
Treatment Position: Supine
Key Rib: Lowest in Group

1. With the patient supine, place one hand on the anterior aspect of the key rib. Flex the patient for pump handle dysfunctions (sidebend the patient for bucket handle dysfunctions) down to the "key" rib.
2. Patient inhales, then exhales deeply. For bucket handle dysfunctions, patient is instructed to reach for their knee on the affected side.
3. The patient is instructed to hold their breath at end-expiratory phase for 3-5 seconds. During this time, the physician adjusts flexion/sidebending to the new restrictive barrier. Physician follows rib shaft into exhalation with his hand during the expiratory phase.
4. Repeat steps 3-4 a total of 3-5 times. Retest for symmetry of motion.

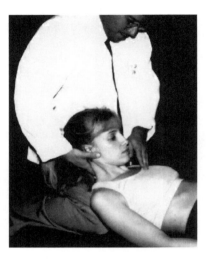

Fig 13.5: Treatment of a Pump-handle dysfunction of Rib 4

Exhalation Dysfunctions
<u>NOTE</u>: There are many different methods used when treating exhalation dysfunctions. Techniques differ slightly. The important concept of these rib treatments is to keep in mind which muscle is being used to correct the dysfunction. This is summarized in table 14.1
Treatment Position: Supine
Key Rib: Top Rib in Group

1. The patient is instructed to place the forearm on the affected side across their forehead with the palm up.
2. The physician grasps the key rib posteriorly at the rib angle.
3. The patient is instructed to inhale deeply while the physician applies an inferior traction on the rib angle.
4. The patient is instructed to hold his breath at full inhalation while performing one of the following isometric contractions for 3-5 seconds:
    ◊ Rib 1:
      Patient raises head directly toward ceiling.
    ◊ Rib 2:
      Patient turns head 30 degrees away from dysfunctional side and lifts head toward ceiling.
    ◊ Ribs 3-5:
      Patient pushes elbow of affected side toward the sternum.
    ◊ Ribs 6-9:
      Push arm anterior.
    ◊ Ribs 10-12:
      Patient adducts arm
5. Repeat step 4 a total of 3-5 times and then retest.

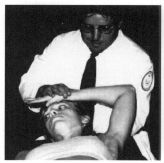
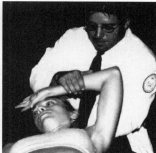
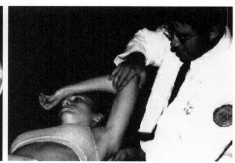

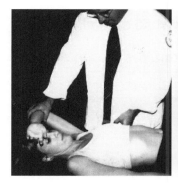
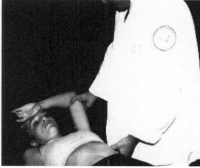

Figures 13.6 a-e
*a: (top left) Treatment of exhalation
  dysfunction of Rib 1.*
*b: (top middle) Treatment of exhalation
  dysfunction of Rib 2.*
*c: (top right) Treatment of exhalation
  dysfunction Ribs 3-5.*
*d: (bottom left) Treatment of
  exhalation dysfunction of Ribs 6-9.*
*e: (bottom right) Treatment of
  exhalation dysfunction of Ribs 11-12.*

Table 14.1 [1 p.711]

Ribs	Muscles
Rib 1	Anterior and Middle Scalenes
Rib 2	Posterior Scalene
Ribs 3-5	Pectoralis Minor
Ribs 6-9	Serratus Anterior
Ribs 10-12	Latissimus Dorsi

Lumbar Spine: Lumbar seated technique
   Positional Diagnosis: L3 ERS$_R$
      Same steps as the lower thoracic spine.

Sacrum:
   Unilateral Sacral Flexion
   Positional Diagnosis: Right USF [1 p.734]
   Treatment Position: Prone
      1. Abduct the patient's right hip to gap the right SI joint. Place your hypothenar eminence on the patient's right ILA.
      2. Ask the patient to inhale and hold his breath, while you push anterior and cephalad on the ILA. Hold for 3-5 seconds.
      3. Direct the patient to exhale while you resist any posterior inferior movement of the sacrum.
      4. Repeat steps two and three 3-5 times and retest.

Unilateral Sacral Extension

Positional Diagnosis: Right USE

Treatment Position: Prone

1. Abduct the patient's right hip to gap the right SI joint. Place your hypothenar eminence on the patient's right sacral sulcus.
2. Ask the patient to exhale and hold their breath, while you push anterior and caudad on the superior sulcus. Hold for 3-5 seconds.
3. Direct the patient to inhale while you resist any anterior superior movement of the sacrum.
4. Repeat steps two and three 3-5 times and retest.

Sacral Torsions:

Positional Diagnosis: L on L (Forward Sacral Torsion)

Treatment Position: Left Lateral Sims Position (lying on left side with face down)

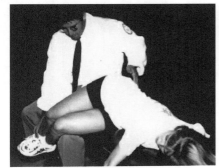

MEMORY TOOL:

Forward sacral torsion patient lies **F**ace down.

1. Patient lies on their left side (*axis side down*) with their torso rotated so that they are face down.
2. Flex patient's hips until motion is felt at the lumbosacral junction.
3. Drop the patient's legs off the table to induce left sidebending and engage a left sacral oblique axis.
4. Ask the patient to lift their legs toward the ceiling against your equal counterforce for 3-5 seconds. Monitor with other hand the right superior pole for posterior movement.
5. Repeat for 3-5 times and then retest for symmetry.

Fig 13.7: Treatment of a L on L, Forward Sacral Torsion

Positional Diagnosis: R on L (Backward Sacral Torsion)

Treatment Position: Left Lateral Recumbent with face up

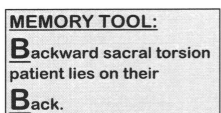

MEMORY TOOL:

Backward sacral torsion patient lies on their **B**ack.

1. Patient lies on their left side (*axis side down*) with his torso rotated so that they are face up.
2. Grasp patient's left arm and pull through to rotate their torso to the right. Flex patient's hips until motion is felt at the lumbosacral junction.
3. Drop the patient's legs off the table to induce left sidebending and engage a left sacral oblique axis.
4. Ask the patient to lift their legs toward the ceiling against your equal counterforce for 3-5 seconds. Monitor with other hand the right superior pole for anterior movement.
5. Repeat for 3-5 times, each time re-engaging the new restrictive barrier, and retest for symmetry of motion.

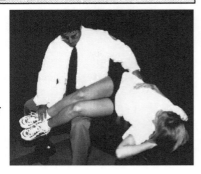

Fig 13.8: Treatment of a R on L, Backward Sacral Torsion.

Innominates:

Positional Diagnosis: Right Innominate Anterior
Treatment Position: Supine

1. Flex patient's right hip and knee until resistance is felt
2. Instruct patient to extend their hip against your counterforce for 3-5 seconds.
3. Wait a few seconds for the tissues to relax, then take up the slack to the new restrictive barrier.
4. Repeat until no restrictive barrier is felt (usually 3-5 times).

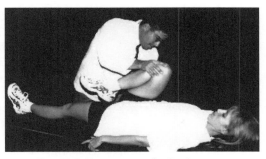

Fig 13.9 Treatment of a Right Innominate Anterior.

Positional Diagnosis: Right Innominate Posterior
Treatment Position: Supine

1. Drop the patient's right leg off the table until resistance is felt. Stabilize the patient's left ASIS with your right hand.
2. Instruct patient to flex his hip against your counterforce for 3-5 seconds.
3. Repeat steps 3 and 4.

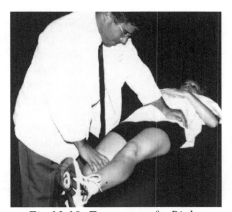

Fig 13.10: Treatment of a Right Innominate Posterior.

Pubic Shears:

Positional Diagnosis: Right Superior Pubic Shear
Treatment Position: Supine

1. Drop the patient's right leg off the table and abduct until resistance is felt. Stabilize the patient's left ASIS with your right hand.
2. Instruct patient to bring his right knee to their left ASIS (flexion and adduction) against your counterforce for 3-5 seconds.
3. Repeat steps 3 and 4.

Positional Diagnosis: Right Inferior Pubic Shear
Treatment Position: Supine

1. Flex and abduct patient's right hip and knee and until resistance is felt. Stabilize the patient's left ASIS with your right hand.
2. Instruct patient to push their right knee to their left foot (extension and adduction) against your counterforce for 3-5 seconds.
3. Repeat steps 3-4.

Upper Extremities:

Positional Diagnosis: Right forearm has restriction of supination (radial head posterior).
Treatment Position: Seated

1. Place your right hand at the distal end of the patient's right forearm and supinate it to initial resistance.
2. Direct the patient to pronate the right forearm against equal resistance supplied through your right hand.
3. Maintain the forces long enough to sense the patient's contractile force at the localized segment or area (usually 3-5 seconds).
4. Both the patient and physician relaxes their forces, the physician takes up the slack to the new point of initial resistance.
5. Repeat for 3-5 times and then recheck findings.

Positional Diagnosis: Right forearm has restriction of pronation (radial head anterior).
Treatment Position: Seated

1. Support the patient's right elbow with your left hand.
2. Place your right hand at the distal end of the patient's right forearm and pronate it to initial resistance.
3. Direct the patient to supinate the right forearm against an equal counterforce supplied through your right hand.
4. Maintain the force for 3-5 seconds, then both the physician and the patient relaxes. The physician then re-engages the new restrictive barrier. Repeat for 3-5 times and then recheck findings.

Lower Extremities

Positional Diagnosis: Right fibular head anterior
Treatment Position: Supine

1. Place your left hand on the lateral side of the patient's foot, cupping the ankle.
2. Invert and dorsi-flex the patient's foot to initial resistance with your right hand grasping bottom of foot.
3. Direct the patient to evert and plantar flex against your isometric counterforce, 3-5 seconds.
4. Relax forces, take up the slack, repeat 3-5 seconds , 3-5 times. Recheck.

Positional Diagnosis: Right fibular head posterior
Treatment Position: Supine

1. Place your left hand on the lateral side of the patient's foot, cupping the ankle.
2. Invert and plantar flex the patient's foot to initial resistance with your right hand grasping bottom of foot.
3. Direct the patient to evert and dorsi-flex against your isometric counterforce, 3-5 seconds.
4. Relax forces, take up the slack, repeat 3-5 seconds , 3-5 times. Recheck.

Chapter **14**
High Velocity Low Amplitude (HVLA)

I. <u>Definition</u>

A **passive, direct technique** which uses high velocity / low amplitude forces to remove motion loss in a somatic dysfunction. After positioning a restricted joint against its restrictive barrier a short (low amplitude) quick (high velocity) thrust is directed to move the joint past the restrictive barrier. HVLA techniques may also be called *thrust techniques, mobilization with impulse treatment.* [1 p.1134]

II. <u>General Procedure</u>:

1. After correct diagnosis of a somatic dysfunction, the physician will move the dysfunctional segment in such a way that it is against its restrictive barrier. This is ideally done by reversing all three planes of motion.
    ◊   For example if a segment was FR_LS_L, the physician would extend, rotate and sidebend the spine to the right (ER_RS_R) until motion is felt at the level of the dysfunctional segment.

    <u>NOTE</u>: Due to the facet orientation and biomechanics in certain regions of the spine it is not always possible to reverse all three planes of motion (i.e. the cervical spine). See specific HVLA techniques for details.

2. The patient then is asked to relax.
    ◊   If the patient is not relaxed, the treatment will fail and the corrective thrust may cause soft tissue damage. The exhalation phase of respiration is the relaxation phase, and the final force is often applied during exhalation. [1 p.664]

3. The physician then uses a short, quick thrust to move the dysfunctional segment through the restrictive barrier. Often a pop or click is heard along with an increase in the range of motion.
    ◊   Be sure to remain against the restrictive barrier before applying the thrust, do not back off before the thrust.

4. Re-evaluate range of motion.

III. <u>Indications and Contraindications</u>

A. <u>Indications</u>

1. <u>Treatment of motion loss in somatic dysfunction</u>. Not ordinarily indicated for treatment of joint restriction due to pathologic changes such as contractures or advanced degenerative joint disease. [1 p.661-2]

B. Absolute contraindications [1, 2, 14, 28]
1. Osteoporosis
2. Osteomyelitis (including Pott's disease)
3. Fractures in the area of thrust
4. Bone metastases
5. Severe rheumatoid arthritis - These patients are at particular risk with cervical manipulation. Rheumatoid arthritis may weaken the transverse ligament of the dens. HVLA manipulation may lead to rupture of this ligament resulting in catastrophic neurologic damage.

C. Relative contraindications [1, 2, 14, 28]
1. Acute whiplash
2. Pregnancy
3. Post-surgical conditions
4. Herniated nucleus propulsis
5. Patients on anticoagulation therapy or hemophiliacs should be treated with great caution to prevent bleeding.
6. Vertebral artery ischemia (positive Wallenberg's test)

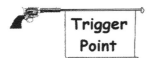

Trigger Point

Know the absolute and relative contraindications for HVLA.

IV. Complications
A. Minor complications:
Most common - Soreness or symptom exacerbation.
B. Major Complications:
Most common overall - *Vertebral artery injury. These problems usually arise with the use of cervical rotatory forces with the neck in the extended position* [1 p.1020]
Most common in the low back - Cauda equina syndrome (very rare).

III. Specific HVLA treatments

A. Cervical
OA FR_LS_R
1.   ͡ ɔ patient supine and the physician at the head of the table.
2. Grasp the patient's head and flex the neck slightly.
3. The MCP joint of the thrusting hand is placed at the base of the occiput.
4. Extend the occiput slightly, make sure that extension is limited to only the OA joint. (NOTE: For an extended OA lesion, flex the head slightly so that flexion is limited to the OA joint).
5. Sidebend the occiput to the left and rotate it to the right to engage the restrictive barrier.
6. Apply a HVLA thrust by translating the occiput to the right. The direction of the thrust should be directed toward the patient's opposite (right) eye.
7. Re-evaluate the range of motion.

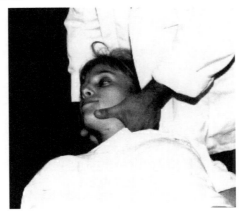

Fig 14.1: Treatment of OA
$FR_LS_R.$

AA rotated right (AAR_R) $\text{AA rotated right (AAR}_R\text{)}$

1. The patient supine and the physician at the head of the table.
2. Grasp the patient's head and flex the neck to approximately 45^0. This will lock out the facets of C2-C7, limiting motion in these segments.
3. Rotate the patient's head to the left engaging the restrictive barrier at the AA.
4. Apply a left rotatory HVLA thrust so that the AA moves through its restrictive barrier.
5. Re-evaluate the range of motion.

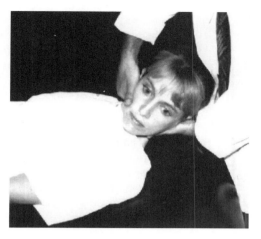

Fig 14.2: Treatment of the AA rotated right.

Typical cervical segments (C2 - C7)

These cervical segments can be treated by using either a sidebending or rotatory thrust. Since these upper segments prefer rotation, typically a rotatory HVLA thrust is used to correct dysfunction. The lower cervical segments prefer sidebending, therefore a sidebending HVLA thrust works well.

As a general rule, in order to limit motion of (lock out) the facets above the dysfunction, the physician must rotate towards the barrier when using a sidebending thrust or sidebend toward the barrier when using a rotational thrust.

C3 FS$_L$R$_L$ Rotational thrust.

1. The patient supine and the physician at the head of the table.
2. Grasp the patient's head and flex the neck slightly.
3. The MCP joint of the thrusting hand is placed at the articular pillar of C3.
4. Extend the neck slightly, make sure that extension is limited to only C3.
5. Sidebend the neck to the left down to C3 to limit motion of (lock) the above facets.
6. Rotate the neck to the right engaging the restrictive barrier at C3.
7. Apply a rotatory HVLA thrust using the left MCP as a fulcrum. The direction of the thrust should be directed toward the patient's opposite (right) eye.
8. Re-evaluate the range of motion.

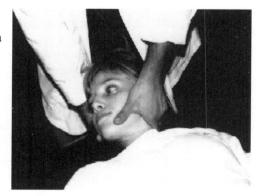

Fig 14.3: Treatment of C3 FR$_L$S$_L$ with a rotational thrust. Remember to sidebend left in order to lock out the facets above C3.

C6 ES$_R$R$_R$ Sidebending thrust.

1. The patient supine and the physician at the head of the table.
2. Grasp the patient's head and flex the neck to the C6 - C7 joint engaging the restrictive barrier.
3. The MCP joint of the thrusting hand is placed at the articular pillar of C6.
4. Rotate the neck to the right to limit motion of (lock) the above facets.
5. Sidebend the neck to the left down to C6 engaging the restrictive barrier.
6. Apply a sidebending HVLA thrust by translating C6 to the right. The direction of the thrust should be directed toward the patient's opposite shoulder.
7. Re-evaluate the range of motion.

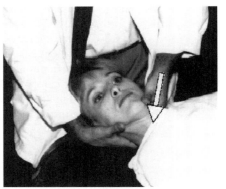

Fig 14.4: Treatment of C6 ES$_R$R$_R$, with a sidebending thrust. Remember to rotate right in order to lock out the facets above C6. The arrow in the diagram demonstrates the direction of the thrust.

B. Thoracics and Ribs

The thoracic segments and ribs can be treated with HVLA in many positions. The position most commonly taught at osteopathic medical schools has been nicknamed the Kirksville Krunch. This technique is easy to understand and versatile. With very little modification of technique the Kirkville Krunch can treat most thoracic and rib dysfunctions. For other types of thoracic HVLA treatments (prone, seated, etc.), please refer to the <u>Foundations of Osteopathic Medicine</u> [1], <u>An Osteopathic Approach to Diagnosis and Treatment</u> [2], or <u>Greenman's Principles of Manual Medicine</u> [14].

When treating a flexed lesion the corrective force will be directed at the dysfunctional segment and the thrust is aimed toward the floor. When treating an extended lesion the corrective thrust is directed at the vertebrae **below** the dysfunctional segment and the thrust is aimed 45^0 cephalad. A neutral lesion is treated the same way as a flexed dysfunction, however sidebend the patient away from you. A purely flexed or extended lesion (no rotation or sidebending) is treated using roughly the same position, except the physician will use a bilateral fulcrum (thenar eminence under one transverse process and a flexed MCP under the other transverse process). Ribs 2-10 can also be treated using the Kirksville Krunch. The difference is that the physician's thenar eminence is under the posterior rib angle of the "key" rib.

T7 FS$_R$R$_R$

1. The patient supine and the physician standing on the left side of the patient (stand on the opposite side of the posterior transverse process).
2. The patient will cross their arm over their chest, so that the superior arm is opposite that of the physician. For simplicity this is referred to as "opposite over adjacent".
3. Place the thenar eminence under the posterior transverse process of the dysfunctional segment.
4. With the other hand flex the patient's torso to the T7 -T8 joint space.
5. Sidebend the patient to the left engaging the restrictive barrier.
6. Have the patient take a deep breath in and exhale.
7. At end exhalation, apply a HVLA thrust straight down toward your fulcrum (thenar eminence).

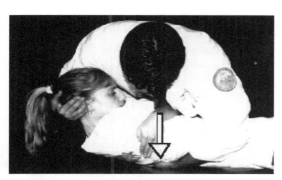

Fig 14.5: Treatment of T7 FR_RS_R. The arrow in the diagram demonstrates the direction of the thrust.

T7 ES$_L$R$_L$

1. The patient supine and the physician standing on the right side of the patient (stand on the opposite side of the posterior transverse process).
2. Patient crosses arms opposite over adjacent.
3. Place the thenar eminence under the posterior transverse process of the vertebrae **below** the dysfunctional segment.
4. With the other hand flex the patient's torso to the T7 - T8 joint space.
5. Sidebend the patient to the right engaging the restrictive barrier.
6. Have the patient take a deep breath in and exhale.
7. At end exhalation, apply a HVLA thrust directed 45^0 cephalad toward your fulcrum (thenar eminence).

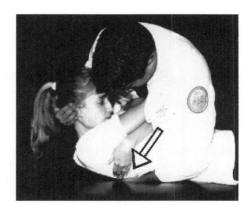

Fig 14.6: Treatment for T7 ES_LR_L. The arrow in the diagram demonstrates the direction of the thrust.

T7 NS$_L$R$_R$

1. The patient supine and the physician standing on the left side of the patient (stand on the opposite side of the posterior transverse process).
2. Patient crosses arms opposite over adjacent.
3. Place the thenar eminence under the posterior transverse process of the dysfunctional segment.
4. With the other hand flex the patient's torso to the T7 - T8 joint space.
5. Sidebend the patient to the right (away from you) engaging the restrictive barrier.
6. Have the patient take a deep breath in and exhale.
7. At end exhalation, apply a HVLA thrust straight down toward your fulcrum (thenar eminence).

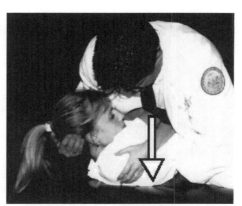

Fig 14.7: Treatment for T7 NS_LR_R. Remember to sidebend the patient away from you to engage the barrier.

Rib 1 Inhalation dysfunction

NOTE: Inhalation dysfunctions of rib one cannot be treated using the Kirksville Krunch.

1. The patient supine and the physician at the head of the table.
2. Sidebend the head and neck to the side of the dysfunctional rib.
3. Rotate the head and neck away.
4. Place 1st MCP on the tubercle of rib 1.
5. Have the patient take a deep breath in and exhale.
6. At end exhalation, apply a HVLA thrust using the 1st MCP as a fulcrum. The direction of the thrust should be medial and caudad.

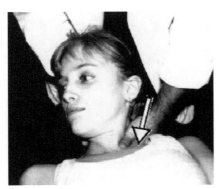

Fig 14.8: Treatment for an Inhalation Dysfunction of Rib 1.

Right Rib 5 Inhalation or Exhalation dysfunction (inhalation or exhalation rib or exhalation or inhalation restriction). Kirksville Krunch treatment type (Range: ribs 2- 10)

1. The patient supine and the physician standing on the left side of the patient (stand on the opposite side of the dysfunctional rib).
2. Patient crosses arms opposite over adjacent.
3. Place the thenar eminence under the posterior rib angle of the "key" rib (see Chapter 3 for further explanation of "key" rib).
4. With the other hand flex the patient's torso and slightly sidebend away from the dysfunctional rib.
5. Have the patient take a deep breath in and exhale.
6. At end exhalation, apply a HVLA thrust straight down toward your fulcrum (thenar eminence).

C. Lumbar Spine

The T10-L5 may be treated with HVLA using the "lumbar roll". Flexion, extension or neutral lesions can all be treated in the same lateral recumbent position. The physician may treat the patient with the posterior transverse up or the posterior transverse process down. For example if L3 was FR_RS_R, the physician can treat the patient in the left lateral recumbent position (posterior transverse process up) or in the right lateral recumbent position (transverse process down). There is only one modification with the patient's position between the two treatments. This modification is italicized in step #6 in the following examples and summarized in table 14.1.

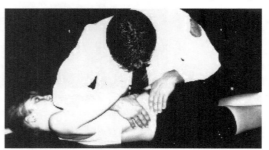

Fig 14.9: Treatment position for a lumbar roll.

Type II (Flexed or Extended) Posterior transverse process up

L3 ER$_R$S$_R$

1. Patient in the left lateral recumbent position (posterior transverse process up).
2. Stand in front of the patient.
3. Flex the patient's legs until you palpate motion at L3.
4. Straighten the patient's inferior leg.
5. Hook the superior foot in the lower legs popliteal fossa.
6. *Pull patient's inferior arm out (toward you) to rotate the torso and down (caudad) to induce left sidebending down to the dysfunctional segment.*
7. Place one arm in the patient's axilla and the other on the patient's iliac crest.
8. Have the patient take a deep breath in and exhale.
9. At end exhalation, apply a HVLA thrust by rotating the patient's pelvis forward and toward the table.
10. Retest the range of motion.

Type II (Flexed or Extended) Posterior transverse process down

L3 ER$_R$S$_R$

1. Patient in the right lateral recumbent position (posterior transverse process down).
2. Stand in front of the patient.
3. Flex the patient's legs until you palpate motion at L3.
4. Straighten the patient's inferior leg.
5. Hook the superior foot in the lower legs popliteal fossa.
6. *Pull patient's inferior arm out (toward you) to rotate the torso and up (cephalad) to induce left sidebending down to the dysfunctional segment.*
7. Place one arm in the patient's axilla and the other on the patient's iliac crest.
8. Have the patient take a deep breath in and exhale.
9. At end exhalation, apply a HVLA thrust by rotating the patient's pelvis forward and toward the table.
10. Retest the range of motion.

NOTE: Flexion or extension can also be added to further engage another barrier. With the patient in the lateral recumbent position, anterior motion of the torso will produce flexion, posterior motion will produce extension.

Type I (neutral dysfunctions) Posterior transverse process up

L3 NS$_L$R$_R$

1. Patient in the left lateral recumbent position (posterior transverse process up).
2. Stand in front of the patient.
3. Flex the patient's legs until you palpate motion at L3.
4. Straighten the patient's inferior leg.
5. Hook the superior foot in the lower legs popliteal fossa.
6. *Pull patient's inferior arm out (toward you) to rotate the torso and up (cephalad) to induce right sidebending down to the dysfunctional segment.*
7. Place one arm in the patient's axilla and the other on the patient's iliac crest.
8. Have the patient take a deep breath in and exhale.
9. At end exhalation, apply a HVLA thrust by rotating the patient's pelvis forward and toward the table.
10. Retest the range of motion.

Type I (neutral dysfunctions) Posterior transverse process down

L3 NS$_L$R$_R$

1. Patient in the right lateral recumbent position (posterior transverse process down).
2. Stand in front of the patient.
3. Flex the patient's legs until you palpate motion at L3.
4. Straighten the patient's inferior leg.
5. Hook the superior foot in the lower legs popliteal fossa.
6. *Pull patient's inferior arm out (toward you) to rotate the torso and down (caudad) to induce right sidebending down to the dysfunctional segment.*
7. Place one arm in the patient's axilla and the other on the patient's iliac crest.
8. Have the patient take a deep breath in and exhale.
9. At end exhalation, apply a HVLA thrust by rotating the patient's pelvis forward and toward the table.
10. Retest the range of motion.

Table 14.1

Lumbar Roll Treatment
Type II Dysfunction:
If treating the patient with the transverse process up => pull the patient's inferior arm down.
If treating the patient with the transverse process down => pull the patient's inferior arm up.
Type I Dysfunction:
If treating the patient with the transverse process up => pull the patient's inferior arm up.
If treating the patient with the transverse process down => pull the patient's inferior arm down.

Chapter **15**
Articulatory Techniques

I. <u>Definition</u>

Articulatory Techniques (also called springing techniques or low velocity / moderate amplitude techniques) are direct techniques that increase range of motion in a restricted joint. The physician engages the restrictive barrier and uses gentle repetitive forces to increase range of motion within that joint. [1 p. 763] Respiratory cooperation and/or muscle energy activation are frequently added to further stretch tight myofascial structures that may limit articular motion.

Post-operative patients and elderly patients find articulatory techniques more acceptable than other vigorous types of direct techniques, since articulating forces are gentle in nature. [1 p.763]

A. <u>Indications</u>:
1. Limited or lost articular motion.
2. Need to increase frequency or amplitude of motion of a body region. For example, the need to increase frequency and amplitude of chest wall motion in a person with respiratory disease.
3. The need to normalize sympathetic activity (rib raising technique). [1 p.450]

B. <u>Contraindications:</u> [1 p.764]
1. Repeated hyper-rotation of the upper cervical spine when positioned in extension may cause damage to the vertebral artery.
2. Acutely inflamed joint especially where the cause of the inflammation may be from an infection or fracture.

C. <u>Typical articulatory procedures</u>
1. Move the affected joint to the limit of all ranges of motion. Once a restrictive barrier is reached slowly and firmly continue to apply gentle force against it.
2. At this time you may use respiratory cooperation or muscle energy activation to further increase myofascial stretch of tight tissues.
3. Return the articulation to its neutral position.
4. Repeat the process several times.
5. Cease repetition of motion when no further response is achieved.

II. <u>Frequently used articulatory techniques</u>

A. <u>Rib Raising</u>
<u>Purpose</u>:
1. Increase chest wall motion
2. Normalize sympathetic activity [1 p.950]
   ◊ Initially rib raising will **increase** sympathetic activity.
   ◊ Prolonged rib raising will **decrease** sympathetic activity.

Rib raising is useful for those patients who have a resistant or noncompliant chest wall, such as a patient with viral pneumonia. **Rib raising will also normalize sympathetic activity**. Rib raising can be done in the seated or supine position. The supine position is described here.

Procedure: [1 p.950]
1. Patient supine.
2. Physician seated at the side of the patient.
3. Place your hands under the patient's thorax, contacting the rib angles with the pads of your fingers.
4. Apply gentle traction.
5. Raise the patients ribs by pushing your fingertips upwards and lowering your forearms (It is easier to push you fingers upward by using your forearm as a lever).

B. Spencer Techniques (Seven Stages of Spencer)

This technique is useful in patients who have developed fibrosis and restriction during a period of inactivity (adhesive capsulitis) following an injury. Such injuries may include a healed rotator cuff tear, or immobilization of the shoulder girdle after a humerus fracture.

The Spencer techniques are performed in 7-stages. In all stages, the patient is in the lateral recumbent position lying with the side of the dysfunctional shoulder up. The physician stands on the side of the table facing the patient, then carefully and slowly moves the upper extremity through the following sequence: [1 pp. 777-780]

Stage I: Extension of the upper extremity with the elbow flexed.

Stage II: Flexion of the upper extremity with the elbow extended.

Stage III: Circumduction with slight compression and the elbow flexed.

Stage IV: Circumduction with traction with the elbow extended.

Stage V: *Broken into 2 parts:*

> **Va:** Abduction with Internal Rotation.

> **Vb:** Adduction and External Rotation.

Stage VI: Abduction and Internal Rotation with the upper extremity behind the back.

Stage VII: Stretching tissues and pumping fluids with the arm extended.

NOTE: The purpose of this technique is to improve motion in the glenohumoral joint, therefore, it is important that the physician limits motion at the scapula by placing his hand on the top of the patient's shoulder. Muscle energy techniques can also be utilized at each of the shoulders' restrictive barriers.

Chapter 16
Special Tests
Glenn S. Fuoco, D.O.

I. Cervical spine
A. Spurling Test (Compression Test)

Narrowing of the neural foramina can cause referred pain into the ipsilateral arm upon compression of the cervical spine, due to nerve root compression. With the patient seated, the physician extends and sidebends the C-spine to the side being tested, and pushes downward on the top of the patient's head. The test is positive if pain radiates into the ipsilateral arm. The pain's distribution can help localize the affected nerve root. [5 p.50-51, 6 p.127, 24 p.411]

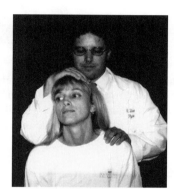

B. Wallenberg's Test

To test for vertebral artery insufficiency, in a supine position the physician flexes the patient's neck, holding it for ten seconds, then extends the neck holding it for ten seconds. The same is done for head and neck rotation to the right and left, head and neck rotation right and left with the neck in the extended position, and in positions that the physician would attempt to mobilize the C-spine. A positive test results when the patient complains of dizziness, visual changes, lightheadedness, or eye nystagmus occurs. [5 p.53-54]

II. Shoulder
A. Adson's Test

This test is for thoracic outlet syndrome and assessment of the subclavian artery. This artery can be compromised with tight scalene muscles, an anomalous cervical rib, somatic dysfunction of the clavicle and upper ribs, or abnormal insertion of pectoralis minor. While monitoring the patient's pulse, the arm is extended at the elbow, the shoulder is extended, externally rotated, and slightly abducted. The patient is then asked to take a deep breath and turn his/her head toward the ipsilateral arm. The test is positive with a severely decreased or absent radial pulse. [1 p.588, 6 p.127, 5 p.122]

B. Apley's scratch test

This test is used to evaluate the range of motion of the shoulder. To test abduction and external rotation, ask the patient to reach behind the head and touch the opposite shoulder. To evaluate internal rotation and adduction, ask the patient to reach in front of the head and touch the opposite shoulder. Next, to further evaluate internal rotation and adduction, instruct the patient to reach behind the back and touch the inferior angle of the opposite scapula. Observe the patient's movement for any asymmetry or any limitations of movement.

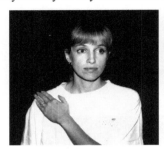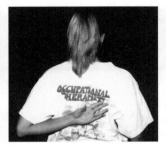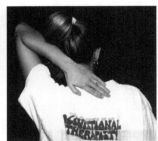

Another way to evaluate range of motion of both shoulders at once is to ask the patient to abduct the arms to 90^0, then supinate the forearms and continue abduction until the hands touch overhead. This will compare bilateral abduction. Next, to test to abduction and external rotation, ask the patient to interlock the hands behind the head and push the elbows posterior. Finally, instruct the patient to place the hands behind the back as high as possible as if to touch the ipsilateral inferior angle of the scapula. [1 p.559, 6 p.21]

C. Drop Arm Test

This test detects tears in the rotator cuff. The patient is instructed to abduct the shoulder to 90^0, and then to slowly lower the arm. A positive test results if the patient cannot lower the arm smoothly, or if the arm drops to the side from 90^0. [1 p.558, 5 p.118]

D. Roos Test

To test for thoracic outlet syndrome, the patient abducts the shoulders to 90^0, externally rotates the shoulders, and flexes the elbows to 90^0. Then, the patient is instructed to slowly open and close both hands for three minutes. The patient should be able to maintain the starting position the entire time. A positive test for TOS results when the arm becomes heavy or there are parasthesias of the hand on the ipsilateral side. [5 p.122]

E. Speed's Test

This test assesses the biceps tendon in the bicipital groove. The patient fully extends the elbow, flexes the shoulder and supinates the forearm. The physician resists the flexion of the shoulder. A positive test occurs with tenderness in the bicipital groove. [5 p.117]

F. Yergason's Test

This test determines the stability of the biceps tendon in the bicipital groove. The patient flexes the elbow to 90^0 while the physician grasps the elbow with one hand and the wrist with the other hand. While pulling downward on the patient's elbow, the physician externally rotates the forearm as the patient resists this motion. A positive test results when pain is elicited as the biceps tendon pops out of the bicipital groove. [1 p.558, 6 p. 32, 5 p.117]

III. Wrist

A. Allen's Test

This test assesses the adequacy of blood supply to the hand by the radial and ulnar arteries. The patient is instructed to open and close the hand being tested several times and then to make a tight fist. The physician occludes the radial and ulnar arteries at the wrist. The patient is then asked to open the hand; the palm should be pale. The physician releases one of the arteries and assesses the flushing of the hand. If it flushes slowly, or not at all, then the released artery is not adequately supplying the hand. This procedure is repeated for the other artery. [1 p.559, 6 p.102-3]

B. Finkelstein Test

To test for tenosynovitis in the abductor pollicis longus and extensor pollicis brevis tendons at the wrist (De Quervain's disease), the patient makes a fist with the thumb tucked inside the fingers. The physician stabilizes the patient's forearm and deviates the wrist ulnarly. A positive test results when the patient feels pain over the tendons at the wrist. [5. p.189: 6 p.76-77]

C. Phalen's Test

This test aides in the diagnosis of carpal tunnel syndrome. The physician maximally flexes the patient's wrist and holds this position for one minute. If a "tingling" sensation is felt in the thumb, index finger, middle and lateral portion of the ring fingers, the test is positive and is indicative of carpal tunnel syndrome. [1 p.559, 6 p.83, 5 p.194]

D. Reverse Phalen's Test (Prayer's test)

Also used in the diagnosis of carpal tunnel syndrome, this test has the patient extend the wrist while gripping the physician's hand. The physician then puts direct pressure on the carpal tunnel. If after one minute, the same symptoms are seen as in Phalen's test, the reverse Phalen's test is positive. [5 p.194]

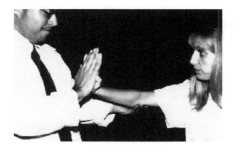

E. Tinel's Test

This test is used in the diagnosis of carpal tunnel syndrome. The physician taps over the volar aspect of the patient's transverse carpal ligament. A positive test will cause tingling or parasthesia into the thumb, index, middle and lateral half of the ring finger. [1 p.559, 5. p.194, 6 p.82]

NOTE: Tinel's test may also be used in the diagnosis of other neuropathies, such as ulnar nerve entrapment at the elbow; and deep peroneal and posterior tibial nerve entrapment at the ankle. [6 p.57, 5 p.484]

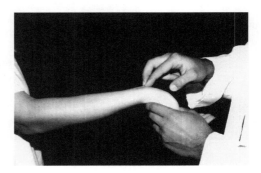

IV. <u>Lumbar spine</u>

A. <u>Hip-drop Test</u>

This test assesses the sidebending ability of the lumbar spine and thoracolumbar junction. With the patient standing, the physician locates the most superior and lateral aspect of the iliac crests. The patient is instructed to bend one knee without lifting the heel from the floor. Normally, the lumber spine should sidebend toward the side contralateral to the bending knee, producing a smooth convexity in the lumbar spine on the ipsilateral side. The ipsilateral iliac crest should drop more than $20\text{-}25^0$. A positive test is indicated by anything less than a smooth convexity in the lumbar spine, or a drop of the iliac crest of less than $20\text{-}25^0$, and alerts the physician to a somatic dysfunction of the lumbar or the thoracolumbar spine.[1 p.497-8]

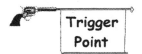
Trigger
Point

The purpose of the Hip drop test is to evaluate sidebending (lateral flexion) of the lumbar spine

B. <u>Straight Leg Raising Test (Lasegue's Test)</u>

This test is used in the evaluation of the lumbar spine, and in sciatic nerve compression. The patient lies supine. The physician grasps the leg being tested under the heel with the hand, and to keep the knee extended, places the other hand on the anterior aspect of the knee. The physician then lifts the leg upward, flexing the hip. The leg is lifted until the patient feels discomfort. Normally, the leg can be raised to about $70\text{-}80^0$ of hip flexion.

If the patient experiences pain, the cause most likely will be due to hamstring tightness or due to problems with the sciatic nerve. Once the patient feels pain upon lifting the leg, the physician lowers the leg just beyond where the pain was felt, and then dorsiflexes the foot (Braggard's Test). This stretches the sciatic nerve. If no pain is elicited, the pain from the leg-raising is probably from tight hamstrings. If pain is felt all the way down the leg, this indicates a sciatic origin. The patient can help localize the source of the pain.[5 p.267, 6 p.256]

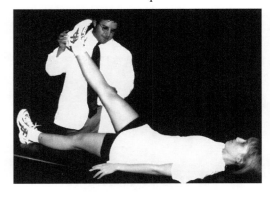
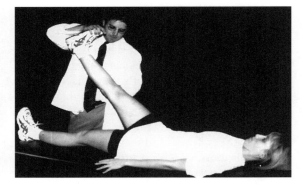

Straight leg raising test   Braggard's test

V. <u>Sacrum and Innominates</u>
A. <u>Seated Flexion Test</u>

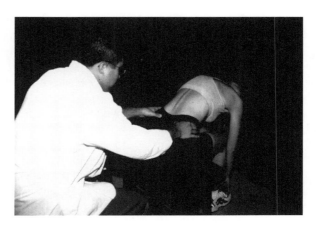

This test assesses **sacroilial motion**. It evaluates somatic dysfunction in the pelvis, most commonly in the sacrum. The patient is seated with both feet flat on the floor. The physician locates the patient's PSIS's and places his thumbs on the inferior notch. The patient is instructed to bend forward and the physician assesses the level of the PSIS's as this motion is completed. A positive test occurs when, at the termination of forward bending, the PSIS's are not level. Somatic dysfunction is present on the side of the superior PSIS. [1 p.498]

B. <u>Standing Flexion Test</u>

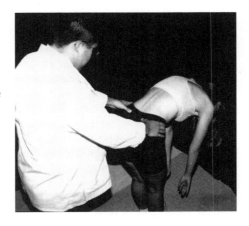

This test assesses **iliosacral motion**. It evaluates the possibility of somatic dysfunction in the leg or pelvis, most commonly the innominate. With the patient standing, the physician locates the patient's PSIS's and places his thumbs on the inferior notch. The patient is instructed to bend forward and the physician assesses the level of the PSIS's as this motion is completed. A positive test occurs when, at the termination of forward bending, the PSIS's are not level. Somatic dysfunction is present on the side of the superior PSIS. [1 p.496]

C. <u>Trendelenberg's Test</u>
This test assesses gluteus medius muscle strength. The physician stands behind the patient. The patient is instructed to pick one of the legs up off the floor. Normally, the gluteus medius muscle should pull up on the unsupported pelvis to keep it level. A positive test occurs when the pelvis falls, which indicates weakness in the gluteus medius muscle. [5 p.323. 6 p.164]

D. <u>Lumbosacral spring test</u> [1 p.615-6]
This test assesses whether or not the sacral base is tilted posterior. With the patient in the prone position, the physician will place the heel of the hand over the lumbosacral junction. Gentle and rapid springing is applied downward onto the lumbosacral junction. The test is positive when there is little or no springing. This is indicative of the sacral base moving posterior.

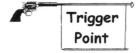
Trigger Point

> **The lumbosacral spring test will be positive in all the dysfunction in which the sacral base moves posterior.**

E. <u>Backward bending test</u> [1 p.616]
This test evaluates sacral somatic dysfunction in the upper arm of the SI joint. The test is positive if a part of the sacral base moves posterior (backward sacral torsion, sacral margin posterior, or a unilateral sacral extension). With the patient prone, the physician places his thumbs on the superior sulci. If asymmetry is present, one side of the sacrum has moved posterior, or the other side has moved anterior. To determine between the two, have the patient prop up on their elbows. This

movement (lumbar extension) causes the sacral base to move anterior. If one side of the sacral base moved anterior, it will move more anterior with lumbar extension and consequently the physician's thumbs will become more symmetrical. However, if part of the sacral base is posterior, it will resist anterior movement with lumbar extension and consequently the physician's thumbs will become more asymmetric.

◊ *If the physician's thumbs become more symmetric with lumbar extension, part of the sacral base moved anterior.*

◊ *If the physician's thumbs become more asymmetric with lumbar extension, part of the sacral base has moved posterior.*

VI. Hips

A. Ober's Test

This test detects a tight iliotibial band. The patient lies on the side opposite the iliotibial band being tested. The physician stands behind the patient and flexes the knee on the side being tested to 90^0, abducts the hip as far as possible, and slightly extends the hip while stabilizing the pelvis to keep the patient from rolling. Slight hip extension is necessary to ensure that the iliotibial band passes directly over the greater trochanter. The physician slowly allows the thigh to fall to the table. The test is positive if the thigh remains in the abducted position, indicating a tight iliotibial band. [5 p.354, 6 p.167]

B. Patrick's Test (FABERE Test)

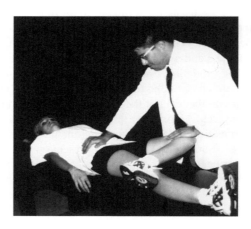

This test is used to assess pathology of the sacroiliac and hip joint, especially osteoarthritis of the hip. The term FABERE indicates the positioning of the hip being tested. Flexion, Abduction, External Rotation, then Extension. The patient's hip is flexed, abducted, and externally rotated into a figure-4 position. Any pain in or around the hip joint indicates general pathology of that hip joint. At this point, the physician places one hand on the contralateral ASIS and the other hand on the knee of the testing leg. Pressure is placed downward on both points, the most important motion being the further extension of the hip. Pain will be accentuated by any arthritic changes in the hip or sacroiliac joint. [1 p.627, 5 p. 343, 6 p.262]

C. Thomas Test

This test assesses the possibility of a flexion contracture of the hip, usually of iliopsoas origin. The patient lies supine and the physician checks for exaggerated lumbar lordosis, common in hip flexion contractures. The physician flexes one hip so that knee and anterior thigh touches the patient's abdomen. If a flexion contracture is not present (photo on right), the patient's opposite leg will remain flat on the table. If present (photo on left), a contracture of the iliopsoas will cause the opposite leg to lift off of the table. [5 p.152, 6 p.155]

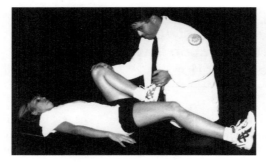 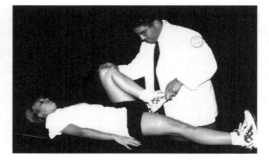

VII. <u>Knee</u>

A. <u>Anterior and Posterior Drawer Tests</u>

These tests are used to assess the anterior and posterior cruciate ligaments. The patient lies supine with the hip flexed to 45^0 and knee flexed to 90^0. The physician sits on the patient's foot of the knee being tested, wraps both hands around behind the tibia, and places one thumb on the medial joint line and one on the lateral joint line. The tibia is then pulled anteriorly (anterior drawer) to test the ACL. If the tibia slides out from under the femur, the test is positive for an ACL tear. Both sides must be compared because some movement may be possible in some patients. The physician then pushes posteriorly on the tibia to check the PCL (posterior drawer). After comparing both knees, the test is positive if the tibia excessively moves backward under the femur. [6 p.186, 5 p.400-2]

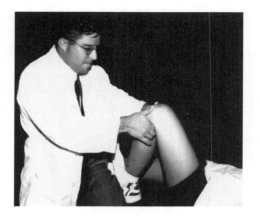

B. <u>Apley's Compression and Distraction Tests</u>

These tests evaluate the meniscus and ligamentous structures of the knee. The patient lies prone and the knee is flexed to 90^0. The compression part of the test is performed with the physician pressing straight down on the heel, and internally and externally rotating the tibia in this position. Pain indicates a meniscal tear. Then, the physician pulls upward (the "distraction" part) on the foot, and internally and externally rotates the tibia. Pain this time indicates ligamentous injury, usually the medial and/or lateral collateral ligaments. [6 p.193, 5 p.413]

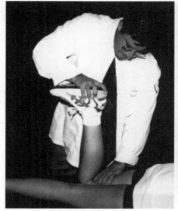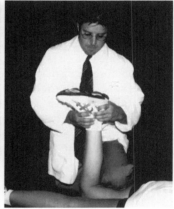

C. <u>Bounce Home Test</u>

This test evaluates problems with full knee extension, usually due to meniscal tears or joint effusions. The patient is supine and the physician grasps the heel. The knee is flexed completely. Then, the knee is allowed to drop into extension. Normally, the knee should "bounce home" into full extension to a sharp end-point, without restriction. The test is positive if extension is incomplete or there is a "rubbery" feel to end-point extension. [1 p.630, 5 p.413, 6 p.194]

D. <u>Lachman's Test</u>

This test also assesses the stability of the ACL and is somewhat more accurate than the drawer tests. The patient lies supine. The physician grasps the proximal tibia with one hand and the distal femur with the other hand. The knee is flexed to about 30^0. The tibia is then pulled forward by the grasping hands. Both sides are compared, and the test is positive if the tibia excessively moves out from under the femur. [1 p.631, 5 p.397]

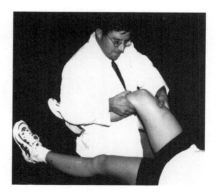

E. McMurray's Test

This test detects tears in the posterior aspect of the menisci. To test the medial meniscus, the patient's knee is fully flexed. The physician's fingers palpate the medial knee joint line. The tibia is then externally rotated and a valgus stress is placed on the knee. Maintaining this position, the knee is then slowly extended. If a palpable or audible "click" is noticed, the test is positive for a posterior tear of the medial meniscus. To test the lateral meniscus, the same procedure is used with internal rotation of the tibia and a varus stress on the knee. [1 p.632, 5 p.413, 6 p.191]

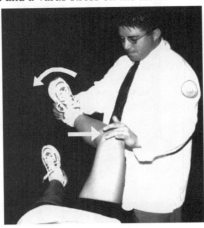 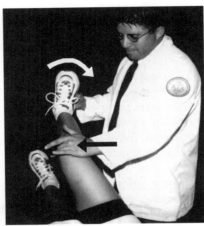

F. Patellar Grind Test

This test assesses the posterior articular surfaces of the patella and the possibility of chondromalacia patellae, commonly seen with lateral femoral patella tracking syndrome. The patient lies supine with knees fully extended and relaxed. The physician pushes the patella distally, then instructs the patient to contract the quadriceps muscles. Any roughness of the articular surfaces will grind, and be palpable and painful when the quadriceps contract and move the patella. The test is positive if the patient feels pain with contraction of the patella. [6 p.194, 5 p.418]

G. Valgus and Varus Stress Tests

These tests are used to assess the stability of the collateral ligaments. With the patient lying supine or sitting on the table, the knee is flexed just enough to unlock it from full extension. The physician stabilizes the ankle with one hand while the other pushes against the knee, first medially then laterally.

Pushing the knee medial (with a **L**ateral force) is the va**L**gus stress test. If there is gapping on the opposite side, then the medial collateral ligament is torn. To test the lateral collateral ligament, the physician pushes the knee laterally (varus stress test), if there is any gaping of the lateral joint line, the test is positive.

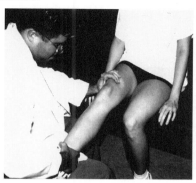 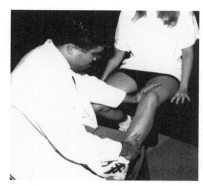

VIII. Ankle

A. Anterior Drawer Test of the Ankle

This test is used to asses the medial and lateral ligaments of the ankle, mainly the anterior talofibular ligament, but also the superficial and deep deltoid ligaments. The patient lies supine. The physician grasps the distal tibia/fibula with one hand, and pulls the foot forward with the other hand grasping the posterior aspect of the calcaneus. The foot should be held in 20^0 of dorsiflexion the entire time. If, after comparing both sides, excessive movement of the talus under the tibia/fibula occurs, then a bilateral injury has occurred to the mentioned ligaments. If there is deviation to one side, then only the ligaments to the opposite side of the foot are damaged. [5 p.480]

1. Which of the following is not an example of a somatic dysfunction?
   A. Acute cholecystitis secondary to gallstones.
   B. Rotator cuff tear secondary to repetitive trauma.
   C. Lumbar strain/sprain.
   D. Osteoarthritis resulting in a decreased range of motion and end range pain.
   E. Adhesive capsulitis.

2. Which one of the following is not a diagnostic characteristic of somatic dysfunction?
   A. Edema.
   B. Temperature change.
   C. Tenderness.
   D. Full range of motion in a joint.
   E. Asymmetry.

3. All of the following are examples of a chronic somatic dysfunction of the right shoulder EXCEPT?
   A. A slight or no increase in temperature of the musculature surrounding the right shoulder.
   B. Asymmetry with noticeable compensation in other areas of the body.
   C. Moist, edematous, erythematous and boggy tissue around the right shoulder.
   D. Restriction with very little or no pain with movement of the right shoulder.

4. In evaluation of a patient with mid-thoracic pain you find that T6 is ER_LS_L (ERS_L). This means that T6 is restricted in?
   A. Flexion, rotation and sidebending to the left in relation to T7.
   B. Flexion, rotation and sidebending to the right in relation to T7.
   C. Flexion, rotation and sidebending to the right in relation to T5.
   D. Extension, rotation and sidebending to the left in relation to T5.
   E. Extension, rotation and sidebending to the right in relation to T5.

5. A point at which a patient can actively move any given joint is defined as?
   A. A physiologic barrier.
   B. A anatomic barrier.
   C. A pathologic/restrictive barrier.
   D. A rotational barrier.
   E. A dysfunctional barrier.

6. While evaluating a patient's upper back pain, you notice that T2 appears to rotated right. Flexing the patient's head down to T2, causes T2 to further rotate to the right. Extending the patient's head causes T2 to return to the neutral position. Which of the following best describes the somatic dysfunction of T2?
   A. ER_RS_R.
   B. FR_RS_R.
   C. ER_RS_L.
   D. FR_RS_L.

7. Which of the following statements concerning Fryette's principle I is true?
   A. Rotation precedes sidebending and occurs to opposite sides.
   B. Sidebending precedes rotation and occurs to opposite sides.
   C. Rotation precedes sidebending and occurs to the same side.
   D. Sidebending precedes rotation and occurs to the same side.

8. Which of the following statements concerning Fryette's principle II is true?
   A. Rotation precedes sidebending and occurs to opposite sides.
   B. Sidebending precedes rotation and occurs to opposite sides.
   C. Rotation precedes sidebending and occurs to the same side.
   D. Sidebending precedes rotation and occurs to the same side.

9. The orientation of the superior facets of the cervical spine is?
   A. Backward and medial.
   B. Backward, upward and lateral.
   C. Backward, upward and medial.
   D. Forward, upward and lateral.
   E. Forward and medial.

10. Motion of vertebral segments along the sagittal plane can best be described as?
    A. Rotation.
    B. Sidebending.
    C. Rotation and sidebending.
    D. Flexion and extension.

11. Motion of vertebral segments along the vertical axis can best be described as?
    A. Rotation.
    B. Sidebending.
    C. Rotation and sidebending.
    D. Flexion and extension

12. Which of the following treatments is correctly matched?
    A. Myofascial release↔Direct technique with passive forces only
    B. Counterstrain↔Indirect technique with passive forces only
    C. Muscle Energy↔Indirect technique with passive forces only
    D. Facilitated Positional Release↔Indirect technique with active forces only
    E. HVLA↔Indirect Technique with passive forces only

13. Which of the following statements concerning muscle contraction is correct?
    A. Isotonic contraction results in the approximation of the muscle's origin and insertion with an increase in tension.
    B. Isometric contraction results in the approximation of the muscle's origin and insertion with an increase in tension.
    C. Isotonic contraction results in an increase in muscle tension <u>without</u> an approximation of origin and insertion.
    D. Isometric contraction results in an increase in muscle tension <u>without</u> an approximation of origin and insertion.
    E. Isotonic contraction results in the approximation of the muscle's origin and insertion with a decrease in tension.

14. Which of the following muscles help elevate the second rib with forced inhalation?
    A. Anterior scalene.
    B. Middle scalene.
    C. Posterior scalene.
    D. Sternocleidomastoid.
    E. Pectoralis minor.

15. Stenosis of the intervertebral foramen between C3 and C4 may effect which nerve root?
    A. C2 nerve root.
    B. C3 nerve root.
    C. C4 nerve root.
    D. C5 nerve root.

16. The primary motion of the occiput on the atlas is?
    A. Flexion/extension.
    B. Sidebending.
    C. Rotation.
    D. Sidebending and rotation.

17. In evaluation of a patient with suboccipital pain you find that his AA is restricted in right rotation. Which of the following statements is true concerning this somatic dysfunction?
    A. The AA will be restricted in left sidebending.
    B. C1 on C2 will be restricted in right sidebending.
    C. The occiput on C1 will be restricted in right sidebending.
    D. C2 on C3 will be restricted in right sidebending.
    E. The occiput on C1 will be restricted in flexion.

18. Which one of the following statements concerning the cervical spine is true?
    A. The uncinate process of the cervical spine is located on the spinous process.
    B. The primary motion of the lower cervical spine is rotation
    C. The primary motion of the lower cervical spine is sidebending.
    D. Decreased translation to the right at C4 suggests that C4 is restricted in left sidebending.
    E. The C2 C3 vertebral unit is responsible for more than 50% of the overall rotation of the cervical spine.

19. All of the following statements concerning the articular pillars are true EXCEPT:
    A. They are used by the osteopathic physician to evaluate cervical motion.
    B. It is the portion of bone located between the superior and inferior facets.
    C. They are located anterior to the cervical transverse processes.
    D. They are also referred to as the lateral masses.

20. Which cervical segment is best evaluated by flexing the neck to 45^0 and rotating the head?
    A. OA.
    B. C1.
    C. C2.
    D. C3.
    E. C4.

21. Using the "rule of three's", the transverse process of T5 can be located:
    A. Half way between the spinous process of T4 and T5.
    B. At the level of the spinous process of T5.
    C. Half way between the spinous process of T5 and T6.
    D. At the level of the spinous process of T6.
    E. At the level of the spinous process of T7.

22. The umbilicus is located at which dermatome?
    A. T4.
    B. T8.
    C. T10.
    D. T12.
    E. L1.

23. The main motion of the thoracic vertebrae is?
    A. Flexion/extension.
    B. Sidebending.
    C. Rotation.
    D. Sidebending and rotation.

24. All of the following are secondary muscles of respiration EXCEPT?
    A. Scalenes.
    B. Pectoralis minor.
    C. External intercostal.
    D. Quadratus lumborum.
    E. Latissimus dorsi.

25. Which of the following groups of ribs are considered false?
    A. Ribs 1-8.
    B. Ribs 7-10.
    C. Ribs 6-10.
    D. Ribs 8-10.
    E. Ribs 7-11.

26. Which of the following groups of ribs are considered atypical?
    A. Ribs 1,2,3,11,12.
    B. Ribs 1,2,3,12.
    C. Ribs 1,3,12.
    D. Ribs 1,2,11,12.
    E. Ribs 1,2,12.

27. A typical rib will have all of the following landmarks EXCEPT?
    A. Tubercle.
    B. Tuberosity.
    C. Head.
    D. Neck.
    E. Angle.

28. A 25 year old male comes to your office complaining of right sided thoracic pain. The pain started after a fall at work approximately one week ago. The severity of the pain has decreased throughout the week however it is still present, especially at maximum inhalation. Advil four times daily seems to decrease the pain. X-rays in your office reveal no fracture. EKG reveals normal sinus rhythm. On examination, you notice that ribs 6-9 on the right are restricted in inhalation, therefore you suspect a rib dysfunction. Which of the following statements correctly describes the diagnosis and treatment?
    A. Inhalation dysfunction and treatment should be directed at rib 9.
    B. Exhalation dysfunction and treatment should be directed at rib 9.
    C. Inhalation dysfunction and treatment should be directed at rib 6.
    D. Exhalation dysfunction and treatment should be directed at rib 6.

29. Which muscle would be used to correct this somatic dysfunction using muscle energy?
    A. Anterior scalene.
    B. Posterior scalene.
    C. Pectoralis minor
    D. Serratus anterior.
    E. Latissimus dorsi.

30. Which one of the following statements concerning ribs 6-9 true?
    A. All of the ribs are considered typical.
    B. All of the ribs are considered typical except rib 9.
    C. All of the ribs are considered atypical.
    D. All of the ribs are considered typical except rib 6.

31. Which one of the following statements concerning the motion of ribs 6-9 is true?
    A. All of the ribs primarily move in a pump-handle motion.
    B. All of the ribs primarily move in a bucket-handle motion.
    C. All of the ribs primarily move in a caliper motion.
    D. All of the ribs primarily move in a pump-handle motion, except rib 9 which moves primarily in a bucket-handle motion.
    E. All of the ribs primarily move in a bucket-handle motion, except rib 6 which moves primarily in a pump-handle motion.

32. Which one of the following statements concerning the thoracic vertebral attachments of ribs 6-9 is true?
    A. Ribs 6-9 attach to T6-T10.
    B. Ribs 6-9 attach to T6-T9.
    C. Ribs 6-9 attach to T5- T9.
    D. Ribs 6-9 attach to T5-T10.

33. Which nerve root exits the intervertebral foramen between the L4 and L5 vertebrae?
    A. L3.
    B. L4.
    C. L5.
    D. S1.

34. A posteriolateral disc herniation of the intervertebral disc of L4/L5 is most likely to compress which nerve root?
    A. L3.
    B. L4.
    C. L5.
    D. S1.

35. All of the following may be seen in a patient with a flexion contracture of the iliopsoas EXCEPT?
    A. A positive Thomas test.
    B. An exaggerated lumbar lordosis.
    C. A decrease in Ferguson's angle.
    D. A somatic dysfunction of the upper lumbar segments.

36. A posterior herniation of the meninges and the nerve roots through a defect in a lumbar vertebral body is called?
    A. Spina bifida occulta.
    B. Spina bifida meningocele.
    C. Spina bifida meningomyelocele
    D. Spondylolisthesis.
    E. Spondylosis.

37. The main motion of the lumbar spine is?
    A. Flexion/extension.
    B. Sidebending.
    C. Rotation.
    D. Sidebending and rotation.

38. A 55 year old male presents to your office with low back pain radiating to his lower extremities. He states that yesterday his feet felt numb and weak, and now this feeling has progressed into his thighs. Neurological examination of his lower extremities reveals: 0/4 deep tendon reflexes; 3/5 muscle strength in his ankle plantar flexors; 3/5 in ankle dorsiflexors; and 3/5 in knee flexors and extensors. You also notice a decreased rectal tone. Which one of the following statements describes the correct course of treatment?
    A. Immediate transportation by EMS to the hospital for neurosurgical evaluation.
    B. Indirect OMT techniques initially to decrease restrictions, followed by direct techniques such as muscle energy, one week later.
    C. Physical modalities, such as ultrasound and electrical stimulation to the low back.
    D. NSAIDS and referral to MRI clinic if pain not improved in one week.
    E. Referral to neurosurgical specialist for evaluation.

39. The anterior displacement of one vertebral body in relation to the one below is known as:
    A. Spondylosis.
    B. Spondylolysis.
    C. Spondylolisthesis.
    D. Spina bifida.
    E. Spinal stenosis.

40. Degenerative changes within the intervertebral disc and ankylosing of adjacent vertebral bodies is known as:
    A. Spondylosis.
    B. Spondylolysis.
    C. Spondylolisthesis.
    D. Spina bifida.
    E. Spinal stenosis.

41. All of the following concerning cauda equina syndrome is true EXCEPT:
    A. It is due to a large central herniation on the cauda equina.
    B. It may result in a weakness in both legs.
    C. It is a surgical emergency.
    D. Paralysis may occur rapidly, but does not usually effect the bladder or rectum.
    E. A decreased sensation to the medial aspect of the thighs and groin, often called "saddle anesthesia" can occur.

42. Which of the structure divides the greater and lesser sciatic foramen?
    A. Sacrotuberous ligament.
    B. Sacrospinous ligament.
    C. Sacroiliac ligament.
    D. Tendon of the obturator internus muscle.
    E. Tendon of the piriformis muscle.

43. Which of the following statements concerning sacral movement is true?
    A. During inhalation the sacral base will move anterior about a transverse axis through S2.
    B. During inhalation the sacral base will move posterior about a transverse axis through S2.
    C. During inhalation the sacral base will move anterior about a transverse axis through S3.
    D. During inhalation the sacral base will move posterior about a transverse axis through S3.
    E. During inhalation the sacral base will move posterior about a transverse axis through S1.

44. Which of the following movements will cause the sacral base to move anterior (sacral flexion)?
    A. Craniosacral flexion.
    B. Counternutation.
    C. Inhalation.
    D. Extension of the lumbar spine.
    E. Weight bearing on the left leg.

45. Which of the following statements concerning sacral counternutation is true?
    A. It occurs during craniosacral flexion as the sacral base moves anterior.
    B. It occurs during craniosacral flexion as the sacral base moves posterior.
    C. It occurs during craniosacral extension as the sacral base moves anterior.
    D. It occurs during craniosacral extension as the sacral base moves posterior.

46. A 32 year old female presents to your office with sacroiliac pain. The pain started 2 days ago after picking up her 3 year old son. On examination you find a positive seated flexion test on the right, L5 NS$_L$R$_R$, her left ILA is shallow, right superior sulcus is deeper, and her lumbar curve is convex to the right. Based on these findings what is the most likely diagnosis?
    A. Right sacral rotation on a right oblique axis (R on R).
    B. Left sacral rotation on a left oblique axis (L on L).
    C. Right sacral rotation on a left oblique axis (R on L).
    D. Left sacral rotation on a right oblique axis (L on R).
    E. A unilateral sacral extension on the right (USE$_R$).

47. Which of the following L5 dysfunctions corresponds with right sacral rotation on a left oblique axis (R on L)?
    A. L5 FR$_L$S$_L$.
    B. L5 NS$_L$R$_R$.
    C. L5 FR$_R$S$_R$.
    D. L5 NS$_R$R$_L$.

48. A 21 year old male is complaining of gluteal pain for 2 days. He states that the pain started after biking several miles. He appears mildly obese and is not physically active. On examination, you notice that his sacral sulci appear shallow. There is a positive lumbosacral spring test. The seated and standing flexion tests are both negative. Based on the information given what is the most likely diagnosis?
    A. Unilateral sacral flexion on the right (USE$_R$).
    B. Bilateral sacral flexion (sacral base anterior).
    C. Unilateral sacral flexion on the left (USE$_L$).
    D. Bilateral sacral extension (sacral base posterior).
    E. Not enough information given to make a diagnosis.

49. A 25 year old medical student is complaining of right sided low back/sacroiliac pain. The pain started one week ago while studying for board exams. On examination, you notice tenderness over the right SI joint, a positive seated flexion test on the right, the sacral sulcus on the right is anterior, while the right ILA is inferior and shallow. Based on the information given what is the most likely diagnosis?
    A. Unilateral sacral extension on the left (USE$_L$).
    B. Unilateral sacral flexion on the left (USF$_L$).
    C. Unilateral sacral extension on the right (USE$_R$).
    D. Unilateral sacral flexion on the right (USF$_R$).
    E. Left sacral rotation on a left oblique axis (L on L).

50. A 30 year old male runner presents with left sided low back pain and left hip pain. The pain started yesterday after a five mile run. It is sharp but does not radiate into the lower extremities. On examination, you notice he has a positive standing flexion test on the left, his left ASIS is inferior, the left PSIS is superior, and his right leg is shorter. Based on the information given what is the most likely diagnosis?
    A. Right posterior innominate.
    B. Left anterior innominate.
    C. Left posterior innominate.
    D. Unilateral sacral flexion on the left (USF_L).
    E. Unilateral sacral extension on the left (USE_L).

51. All of the following can cause a positive seated flexion test on the right EXCEPT:
    A. Unilateral sacral extension on the right (USE_R).
    B. Unilateral sacral flexion on the right (USF_R).
    C. Left sacral rotation on a left oblique axis (L on L).
    D. Right sacral rotation on a right oblique axis (R on R).
    E. Sacral margin posterior on the right.

52. Which of the following will produce a deep sacral sulcus on the right?
    A. Unilateral sacral extension on the right (USE_R).
    B. Unilateral sacral flexion on the right (USF_R).
    C. Right sacral rotation on a left oblique axis (R on L).
    D. Right sacral rotation on a right oblique axis (R on R).
    E. Unilateral sacral flexion on the left (USF_L).

53. Which of the following findings is present in a left innominate anterior rotation?
    A. PSIS inferior on the left.
    B. PSIS superior on the right.
    C. PSIS superior on the left.
    D. ASIS superior on the left.
    E. PSIS and ASIS posterior on the left.

54. All of the following muscles make up the rotator cuff EXCEPT:
    A. Supraspinatus.
    B. Infraspinatus.
    C. Teres major.
    D. Teres minor.
    E. Subscapularis.

55. Which one of the following muscles is the primary internal rotator of the humerus?
    A. Teres minor.
    B. Subscapularis.
    C. Infraspinatus.
    D. Pectoralis minor.
    E. Deltoid.

56. Which one of the following statements is true concerning the radial artery?
    A. It branches directly from the profunda (deep) brachial artery and accompanies the radial nerve in the posterior course of the radial groove.
    B. It branches directly from the axillary artery to supply the lateral aspect of the forearm.
    C. It branches directly from the axillary artery to supply the medial aspect of the forearm.
    D. It forms most of the deep palmar arch of the hand.

57. What is the correct sequence of nerve divisions leaving the spinal cord to form the brachial plexus?
    A. Roots, trunks, branches, cords, divisions.
    B. Roots, divisions, trunks, cords, branches.
    C. Roots, trunks, cords, branches, divisions.
    D. Roots, cords, trunks, branches, divisions.
    E. Roots, trunks, divisions, cords, branches.

58. Which of the following nerves only carries fibers from the C5 nerve root?
    A. Musculocutaneous
    B. Lateral Pectoral
    C. Suprascapular
    D. Long Thoracic
    E. Dorsal scapular

59. An injury to the C5 nerve root will most likely cause partial paralysis in which group of muscles?
    A. The finger abductors.
    B. The wrist extensors.
    C. The elbow flexors.
    D. The forearm pronators.
    E. The wrist flexors.

60. Upper arm paralysis caused by an injury to the C5 and C6 nerve roots usually during childbirth is also known as?
    A. Klumpke's palsy.
    B. Erb-Duchenne's palsy.
    C. Stick palsy .
    D. Long thoracic nerve palsy.
    E. Bell's palsy.

61. Decreased sensation over the medial aspect of the forearm associated with weak adduction of the wrist suggests pathology in which nerve root?
    A. C5.
    B. C6.
    C. C7.
    D. T1.

62. Which of the following findings is most likely to be present in a patient that suffers from a lower motor neuron injury affecting the C5 and C6 nerve roots?
    A. A decreased biceps reflex.
    B. An increased triceps reflex.
    C. An increased biceps reflex.
    D. Decreased sensation over the ring and little fingers.
    E. Decreased sensation over the medial epicondyle.

63. An 80 year old female suffered a stroke several weeks prior. After rehabilitation, she has a full range of motion in her left arm against gravity with no resistance. You would grade the muscle strength in her left arm as:
    A. 0/5.
    B. 1/5.
    C. 2/5.
    D. 3/5.
    E. 4/5.

64. A 31 year old female presents to your office with neck pain following a motor vehicle accident two days ago. She states that her pain is a dull ache on the right side of her neck that radiates into her arm. On examination, you notice a right anterior scalene tenderpoint and positive Adson's and Roos tests. Neurological exam reveals no sensory deficits, 5/5 muscle strength, and normal deep tendon reflexes. Your most likely diagnosis is?
    A. Bicipital tenosynovitis
    B. A rotator cuff tear.
    C. Thoracic outlet syndrome.
    D. Supraspinatus tendonitis.
    E. Herniated nucleus propulsis of the cervical spine.

65. Thoracic outlet syndrome is due to compression of the neurovascular bundle (subclavian artery and vein and brachial plexus). This compression can occur in all of the following locations EXCEPT:
    A. Between the anterior and middle scalene muscles.
    B. Between the middle and posterior scalenes.
    C. Between the pectoralis minor and the upper ribs.
    D. Between the clavicle and the first rib.

66. Humeral dislocation is most likely to occur in which position?
    A. Inferior and posterior.
    B. Anterior and inferior.
    C. Superior and anterior.
    D. Superior and anterior.
    E. Posterior.

67. A 21 year old right-handed minor league pitcher presents to your office with right shoulder pain. The pain has increased gradually over the past month, and worsens with pitching. Ice and ibuprofen seem to decrease the pain. On examination, you notice tenderness at the tip of the acromion. He has full range of motion of the right shoulder, but has pain with abduction, especially from $60^0 - 120^0$. He has a positive drop arm test. Neurological examination of the upper extremity is within normal limits. The most likely cause of his pain is?
    A. Bicipital tenosynovitis.
    B. Adhesive capsulitis.
    C. Supraspinatus tendonitis.
    D. Complete rupture of the supraspinatus tendon.
    E. A cervical rib.

68. Winging of the scapula can be caused by damage to which nerve?
    A. Dorsal scapular.
    B. Long thoracic.
    C. Suprascapular.
    D. Lower subscapular.
    E. Thoracodorsal.

69. Which of the following carpal bones is located most medially?
    A. Scaphoid
    B. Trapezoid
    C. Lunate
    D. Capitate
    E. Hamate

70. All of the following muscles of the hand are innervated by the median nerve EXCEPT:
    A. Abductor pollicis brevis.
    B. Adductor pollicis.
    C. Opponens pollicis.
    D. First and second lumbricals.

71. Pronators of the forearm are primarily innervated by which one of the following nerves?
    A. Median.
    B. Ulnar.
    C. Radial.
    D. Musculocutaneous.

72. A 15 year old female presents to your office with left wrist and elbow pain. The pain started one week ago. On examination, you notice tenderpoints at the elbow and wrist, she has an increased carrying angle on her left side. Her wrist appears to be restricted in abduction. And X-rays show no evidence of any fractures. Assuming she has somatic dysfunction at her left elbow, which choice is the most likely diagnosis?
    A. Posterior radial head.
    B. Anterior radial head.
    C. Adduction of the ulna.
    D. Abduction of the ulna.

73. Which of the following movements will cause the radial head to glide anterior?
    A. Pronation of the forearm.
    B. Supination of the forearm.
    C. Flexion of the wrist.
    D. Extension of the wrist.
    E. Extension of the elbow.

74. A 35 year old female presents with numbness and tingling over the palmar surface of her right thumb. She states symptoms often radiates into her first and middle fingers. It started six months ago and has gotten increasingly worse. Tylenol and Advil seem to alleviate the symptoms somewhat. On examination, you notice a decreased sensation at the pads of the first and middle fingers, and decreased grip strength of the right hand. Tinel's test at the wrist is positive. The most likely cause of her pain is?
    A. Thoracic outlet syndrome.
    B. Syphilis.
    C. A scaphoid fracture.
    D. Carpal tunnel syndrome.

75. Which nerve is most likely to be effected in the above question?
    A. Median nerve.
    B. Ulnar nerve.
    C. Radial nerve.
    D. Musculocutaneous nerve.

76. Tennis elbow is often associated with tenderness at which anatomical landmark?
    A. The olecrenon.
    B. The bicipital aponeurosis.
    C. The lateral epicondyle.
    D. The medial epicondyle.
    E. The humeral condyles

77. Wrist drop deformity is associated with damage to which one of the following structures?
    A. Median nerve.
    B. Wrist flexor muscles.
    C. Flexor retinaculum.
    D. Ulnar nerve.
    E. Radial nerve.

78. The origin of the brachial artery is located at:
    A. The superior border of pectoralis minor.
    B. The lateral border of the first rib.
    C. The superior border of teres minor.
    D. The inferior border of teres minor.
    E. The inferior/lateral border of the clavicle.

79. All of the following is associated with cubitus valgus EXCEPT:
    A. Abduction of the ulna.
    B. An increased carrying angle.
    C. Adduction of the wrist.
    D. A posterior radial head.

80. Which muscle is considered to be the primary flexor of the hip?
    A. Gluteus medius.
    B. Gluteus maximus.
    C. Iliopsoas.
    D. Quadriceps.
    E. Hamstrings.

81. Which structure prevents hyperextension of the knee?
    A. The posterior cruciate ligament.
    B. The anterior cruciate ligament.
    C. The medial meniscus.
    D. The medial collateral ligament.
    E. The lateral collateral ligament.

82. A patient with a herniated nucleus propulsus compressing the L5 nerve root will have the greatest loss of strength in which muscle?
    A. Anterior tibialis.
    B. Extensor hallicus longus.
    C. Iliopsoas.
    D. Adductors and quadriceps.

83. You would expect the above patient to have the greatest decreased sensation at which anatomical structure?
    A. Lateral malleolus.
    B. Medial malleolus.
    C. Big toe.
    D. Knee

84. An insult to the knee often referred to as "O'Donahue's triad", "the terrible triad", or "the unhappy triad" results in injury to which of the following structures?
   A. The medial meniscus, the anterior cruciate ligament and the lateral collateral ligament.
   B. The lateral meniscus, the anterior cruciate ligament and the medial collateral ligament.
   C. The medial meniscus, the anterior cruciate ligament and the lateral meniscus.
   D. The medial meniscus, the anterior cruciate ligament and the medial collateral ligament.
   E. The medial meniscus, the posterior cruciate ligament and the lateral collateral ligament.

85. All of the following is associated with a posterior fibular head dysfunction EXCEPT:
   A. It often occurs following a supination ankle sprain.
   B. The foot will appear more supinated on the affected side.
   C. There will be a restriction in posterior glide of the fibular head.
   D. Dorsiflexion of the ankle will be restricted on the affected side.

86. The condition in which there is a decrease in the angle between the neck and the shaft of the femur is called:
   A. Coxa valga.
   B. Coxa vara.
   C. Genu varum.
   D. Genu valgum.
   E. A decreased Q angle.

87. A decreased Q angle is associated with which one of the following conditions?
   A. Genu valgum.
   B. Lateral femoral patella tracking syndrome.
   C. A bow-legged appearance.
   D. Coxa vara.

88. All of the following is true concerning lateral femoral patella tracking EXCEPT:
   A. It is associated with accelerated wearing on the posterior surface of the patella.
   B. It occurs most often in women.
   C. It is associated with a positive Lachman's test.
   D. The patient may complain of deep knee pain that worsens when climbing stairs.

89. The treatment for lateral femoral patella tracking is focused on strengthening which muscle(s)?
   A. Rectus femoris.
   B. Vastus lateralis.
   C. Vastus medialis.
   D. The hamstrings.
   E. Gastrocnemius.

90. An injury to a ligament, in which a portion of the fiber is disrupted, is referred to as which of the following types of sprains?
   A. First degree sprain.
   B. Second degree sprain.
   C. Third degree sprain.
   D. Fourth degree sprain.

91. Which compartment of the lower leg is most often effected in "compartment syndrome"?
   A. The lateral compartment.
   B. The anterior compartment.
   C. The deep posterior compartment.
   D. The superficial posterior compartment.

92. All of the following are lateral stabilizers of the ankle (ligaments that prevent excessive supination) EXCEPT:
    A. The anterior talofibular ligament.
    B. The calcaneonavicular ligament.
    C. The calcaneofibular ligament.
    D. The posterior talofibular ligament.

93. The ligament most often injured in supination ankle sprains is:
    A. The anterior talofibular ligament.
    B. The calcaneonavicular ligament.
    C. The calcaneofibular ligament.
    D. The posterior talofibular ligament.

94. The ankle is most stable in which one of the following positions?
    A. Supination.
    B. Inversion.
    C. Plantar flexion
    D. Dorsiflexion.

95. A type II supination ankle sprain implies that there is injury to which of the following ligaments?
    A. The anterior talofibular ligament.
    B. The anterior talofibular and the calcaneofibular ligament.
    C. The anterior talofibular the calcaneofibular, and the posterior talofibular ligament.
    D. The posterior talofibular and the calcaneofibular ligament.
    E. The deltoid ligament.

96. A fracture of the proximal fibular head is most likely to effect which nerve?
    A. Sciatic nerve.
    B. Common fibular nerve.
    C. Tibial nerve.
    D. Sural nerve.
    E. Femoral nerve.

97. All of the following are components of the lateral longitudinal arch EXCEPT:
    A. Navicular.
    B. Cuboid.
    C. Fourth metatarsal.
    D. Fifth metatarsal.
    E. Calcaneus.

98. All of the following are components of the primary reciprocal membrane EXCEPT:
    A. The CNS.
    B. The CSF.
    C. The dural membranes.
    D. The cranial bones.

99. All of the following are anatomical - physiological elements that make up the PRM EXCEPT:
    A. The inherent motility of the brain and spinal cord.
    B. The fluctuation of the CSF.
    C. Mobility of the intracranial and intraspinal membranes.
    D. The immobility of the sphenobasilar synchondrosis.
    E. The involuntary mobility of the cranial bones.

100. The dura mater has firm attachments to all of the following structures EXCEPT:
    A. Foramen magnum.
    B. C2.
    C. C3.
    D. C7.
    E. S2.

101. All of the following are considered midline bones EXCEPT:
    A. Sphenoid.
    B. Occiput.
    C. Parietal.
    D. Vomer.
    E. Ethmoid.

102. Flexion of the midline bones will cause:
    A. Internal rotation of the paired bones and a decrease in the anterio-posterior diameter of the cranium.
    B. External rotation of the paired bones and a decrease in the anterio-posterior diameter of the cranium.
    C. Internal rotation of the paired bones and an increase in the anterio-posterior diameter of the cranium.
    D. External rotation of the paired bones and an increase in the anterio-posterior diameter of the cranium.

103. All of the following is associated with craniosacral flexion EXCEPT:
    A. Deviation of the SBS cephalad.
    B. Counternutation.
    C. Sacral extension about a transverse axis through S2.
    D. A decreased width of the cranium.
    E. External rotation of the temporal bones.

104. While palpating a patient's cranium you notice that the greater wing of the sphenoid feels more superior on the right than the left. You also notice that the occiput is rotated in the opposite direction. This best describes which type of strain pattern?
    A. A right torsion.
    B. A left torsion.
    C. A left lateral strain.
    D. Sidebending and rotation to the left.
    E. Sidebending and rotation to the right.

105. Which of the following strains can be considered physiologic if it does not interfere with the flexion/extension components of the mechanism?
    A. A vertical strain.
    B. A lateral strain.
    C. Compression at the SBS.
    D. A torsion.

106. Which of the following strains is associated with an absent C.R.I.?
    A. A vertical strain.
    B. A lateral strain.
    C. Compression at the SBS.
    D. A torsion.
    E. sidebending and rotation strain.

107. Which of the following cranial somatic dysfunctions may result in tinnitus?
    A. Sphenoid restriction interfering with CN X.
    B. Temporal restriction interfering with CN VIII.
    C. Ethmoid restriction interfering with CN I.
    D. Temporal restriction interfering with CN VII.

108. Somatic dysfunction in all of the following may cause diplopia EXCEPT:
    A. The sphenoid.
    B. The temporal.
    C. The occiput.
    D. CN III.
    E. CN VI.

109. Dysfunction of which cranial nerve can cause symptoms similar to Tic Douloureux?
    A. CN V V_1.
    B. CN V V_2.
    C. CN V V_3.
    D. CN III.
    E. CN VII.

110. Which one of the following cranial nerves exit the foramen rotundum?
    A. A. CN V V_1.
    B. CN V V_2.
    C. CN V V_3.
    D. CN III.
    E. CN VII.

111. All of the following cranial nerves exit the jugular foramen EXCEPT:
    A. CN IX.
    B. CN X.
    C. CN XI.
    D. CN XII.

112. Somatic dysfunction of C2 may alter the function of which cranial nerve?
    A. CN IX.
    B. CN X.
    C. CN XI.
    D. CN XII.

113. All of the following are relative or absolute contraindications to craniosacral therapy EXCEPT:
    A. An acute intracranial bleed.
    B. A skull fracture.
    C. Traumatic brain injury.
    D. A migraine headache.
    E. A history of seizure disorder.

114. All of the following are true concerning stimulation of sympathetic chain ganglia at T3 EXCEPT:
    A. It will cause dilation of the pupil.
    B. It will cause an increase in heart rate.
    C. It will cause bronchodilation.
    D. It will stimulate lacrimal secretion.

MATCHING
  A. Venous sinus technique.
  B. CV4 technique.
  C. Vault hold.
  D. Temporal rocking.
  E. V spread.

_A_ – 115. Enhances venous blood flow through the venous sinuses.
_E_ – 116. Separates restricted or impacted sutures.
_D_ – 117. A valuable technique to help TMJ dysfunction.
_C_ – 118. Addresses strains at the SBS.
_B_ – 119. Enhances the amplitude of the C.R.I.

120. Which of the following vertebral segments will have the least effect on cardiac function?
  A. T3.
  B. T7.
  C. T4.
  D. OA.
  E. AA.

121. All of the following are true concerning vagus nerve stimulation EXCEPT:
  A. It will cause a decrease in contractility of the heart.
  B. It will cause pupillary constriction.
  C. It will cause an increase in gastric motility.
  D. It will cause bladder wall contraction.

122. All of the following are true concerning a facilitated segment EXCEPT:
  A. Less afferent stimulation is required to trigger a discharge of efferent neurons.
  B. Once established, it can be sustained by normal CNS activity.
  C. Has an increased efferent output.
  D. Usually caused by a decrease in afferent input.
  E. It has a low threshold of excitation.

123. A 15 year old male presents to your office with an acute asthmatic exacerbation. Viscero-somatic changes associated with asthma can be seen at which spinal level?
  A. C2-C7.
  B. T2-T6.
  C. T5-T10.
  D. T9-T11.
  E. T12-L2.

124. Treatment of the OA and AA may effect all of the following visceral structures EXCEPT:
  A. Prostate.
  B. Kidney.
  C. Ureter.
  D. Transverse colon.
  E. Ovaries.

125. Which of the following will result from sympathetic stimulation?
  A. Increase in gastric motility.
  B. Diarrhea.
  C. Increase in respiratory rate.
  D. Lacrimation.
  E. Miosis.

126. A 42 year old obese female presents to your office with right upper quadrant pain. Pain radiates to the tip of the right scapula. On examination, you notice a positive Murphy's sign. You suspect acute cholecystitis. At which vertebral level would you expect to find somatic changes?
    A. T1-T4.
    B. T6-T9.
    C. T9-T11.
    D. T11-L2.

127. Obstruction of a ureter from a calcium oxalate stone resulting in hydronephrosis and acute pyelonephritis may effect all of the following autonomic nerves EXCEPT:
    A. Vagus.
    B. Pelvic splanchnic.
    C. Sympathetic chain ganglia of T12-L1.
    D. Sympathetic chain ganglia of L4-L5.
    E. Sympathetic chain ganglia of T10-T11.

128. A viscero-somatic reflex resulting from a right colon cancer would be associated with somatic changes at which spinal segment?
    A. T1-T5.
    B. T6-T8.
    C. T9-T11.
    D. T12-L2.

129. Stimulation of sympathetic chain ganglia may cause all of the following EXCEPT:
    A. Digestion.
    B. Ejaculation.
    C. Vasodilation of blood vessels supplying skeletal muscle.
    D. Diaphoresis.
    E. Increased heart rate.

130. Which of the following spinal segments may alter the parasympathetic innervation to the appendix?
    A. AA.
    B. C7.
    C. T9-T12.
    D. T12-L1.
    E. S2-S4.

131. Sympathetic innervation to the liver is through which one of the following ganglia?
    A. Superior cervical.
    B. Celiac.
    C. Superior mesenteric.
    D. Inferior mesenteric.
    E. Pelvic mesenteric.

132. A 75 year old male presents to your office with difficulty urinating. You suspect a prostate problem. Treatment to which one of the following spinal segments may calm the sympathetic influence on the prostate?
    A. T5.
    B. T8.
    C. T12.
    D. L1.
    E. S2.

133. Restriction of the occipitomastoid suture at the jugular foramen may cause all of the following visceral dysfunctions EXCEPT:
    A. Gastritis.
    B. Diarrhea.
    C. Bradycardia.
    D. Stress incontinence.
    E. Irritable bowel syndrome.

134. An increase in the sympathetic tone of the abdominal cavity will result in all of the following EXCEPT:
    A. An increase in gluconeogenesis.
    B. An increase in pancreatic secretion.
    C. A decrease in gastric motility.
    D. A decrease in GI absorption.

135. Which of the following will influence the parasympathetic supply to the ovaries?
    A. The vagus.
    B. T12-L2.
    C. T9-T11.
    D. S2-S4.

136. A 25 year old female presents to your office with dysmenorrhea. Viscero-somatic reflex changes associated with uterine dysfunction may be at which spinal level?
    A. AA.
    B. C7.
    C. T12.
    D. L4.

137. A 45 year old male with paroxysmal hypertension secondary to an adrenal pheochromocytoma may have somatic changes at which spinal level?
    A. OA.
    B. T8.
    C. T10.
    D. T12.
    E. L2.

138. Parasympathetic stimulation to the head and thorax may cause all of the following EXCEPT:
    A. Lacrimation.
    B. Bradycardia.
    C. Miosis.
    D. Bronchodilation

139. Sympathetic stimulation of segments T10-L2 may cause which one of the following reactions?
    A. Ejaculation.
    B. Erection.
    C. Bradycardia.
    D. Increased lymphatic drainage of the lower extremities.
    E. Pancreatic secretion.

140. All of the following are true concerning Chapman's reflex points EXCEPT:
    A. They are thought to represent viscero-somatic reflexes.
    B. They are discretely palpable nodules 2-3 mm in diameter.
    C. Upon compression they can give rise to a characteristic referred pain, tenderness or autonomic phenomena.
    D. They are used more for diagnosis than treatment in current clinical practice.

141. Which one of the following Chapman's reflex points is associated with the appendix?
    A. The tip of the eleventh right rib.
    B. The tip of the twelfth right rib.
    C. The spinous process of L1.
    D. The spinous process of L2.
    E. The spinous process of T12.

142. All of the following statements are true concerning tenderpoints EXCEPT:
    A. They are hypersensitive points in myofascial tissue.
    B. They act as a treatment monitor for counterstrain.
    C. They often refer pain when compressed.
    D. They are painful when compressed.

143. When performing indirect myofascial release, which barrier is engaged?
    A. Pathologic
    B. Restrictive
    C. Anatomic
    D. Physiologic
    E. Both A and B

144. Which of the following is **NOT** an appropriate endpoint of myofascial release treatment?
    A. A warming of the region treated
    B. Restoration of symmetry
    C. "Melting" of the restrictive barrier
    D. A sufficient amount of time has passed and no release was felt
    E. All are appropriate

145. Which of the following is **NOT** a contraindication for treatment utilizing myofascial release?
    A. Febrile bacterial infection
    B. Peripheral edema
    C. Osseous fracture
    D. Advanced stage cancer
    E. Traumatic disruption of internal organs

146. Which of the following structures is considered to be a physiologic diaphragm?
    A. Hard and soft pallate
    B. Tentorium cerebelli
    C. Greater omentum
    D. Broad ligament of the uterus
    E. Mediastinum

147. Which of the following is **INCORRECTLY** matched according to the common compensatory pattern described by Zink?
    A. OA → Left
    B. Cervicothoracic → Right
    C. Lumbosacral → Right
    D. All are correctly matched
    E. None are correctly matched

148. What percentage of tenderpoints are likely to be "maverick"?
    A. 1%
    B. 5%
    C. 7%
    D. 10%
    E. 15%

149. When fine tuning position for a counterstrain technique, what is the minimum acceptable reduction of pain?
    A. 50%
    B. 60%
    C. 70%
    D. 85%
    E. 95%

150. What region is associated with the greatest number of "maverick" tenderpoints?
    A. Cervical spine
    B. Thoracic spine
    C. Lumbar spine
    D. Ribs
    E. Pelvis

151. When utilizing facilitated positional release to a superficial muscle, which is performed first?
    A. Application of traction
    B. Application of compression
    C. Shortening of the muscle
    D. Straightening of the AP spinal curves
    E. Fine tuning the position

152. Which of the following is **NOT** correctly matched?
    A. Counterstrain → Hold 90 seconds
    B. Facilitated positional release → Hold 30 seconds
    C. Posterior cervical tenderpoint → Tip of spinous process
    D. Posterior rib tenderpoint → Angle of rib
    E. All are correctly matched

153. Which of the following is the correct location for the iliacus tenderpoint?
    A. On the ASIS
    B. 1 cm lateral to the ASIS
    C. 3 cm medial to the ASIS
    D. 5 cm lateral to the ASIS
    E. 7 cm medial to the ASIS

154. Which of the following is a necessary component for any successful muscle energy treatment?
    A. Reciprocal inhibition
    B. Postisometric relaxation
    C. Responsive patient
    D. Direct treatment of pathologic barrier
    E. Holding the position for 90 seconds

155. Which is true regarding the localization of forces used in a direct muscle energy technique?
    A. Applied force must address a single plane of motion
    B. The counterforce used by the physician should be greater than the force applied by the patient
    C. The counterforce used by the physician should be less than the force applied by the patient
    D. A few seconds after the patient relaxes, the physician takes up the slack in all planes of motion
    E. None of the above are correct

156. Which joint is treated by the use of rotational force <u>only</u>?
    A. OA
    B. AA
    C. C3
    D. T2
    E. Posterior radial head

157. Which of the following segments is **NOT** treated by inducing the motion of the patient's head?
    A. OA
    B. C2
    C. C7
    D. T6
    E. 2nd rib exhalation dysfunction

158. Which muscle is used to treat an exhalation dysfunction of rib 11 with a muscle energy technique?
    A. Serratus anterior
    B. Serratus posterior
    C. Quadratus lumborum
    D. Ilicostalis
    E. Latissimus dorsi

159. In which patient would muscle energy techniques be contraindicated?
    A. 23 year old paraplegic
    B. 6 year old healthy child
    C. 76 year old healthy man
    D. 38 year old female immediately post MI
    E. 45 year old male with GERD

160. Which of the following is **FALSE** regarding HVLA?
    A. The techniques are passive
    B. The techniques are indirect
    C. The techniques involve a short, quick thrust
    D. The thrust is usually performed during exhalation
    E. A pop or click may be heard

161. Which of the following is **NOT** an absolute contraindication for HVLA?
    A. Fracture
    B. Rheumatoid arthritis
    C. Osteoporosis
    D. Tenosynovitis
    E. Pott's disease

162. Which of the following is **NOT** a relative contraindication for HVLA?
    A. Herniated nucleus pulposis
    B. Pregnancy
    C. Vertebral artery insufficiency
    D. Hemophila A
    E. Scoliosis

163. Which is true of low velocity / moderate amplitude techniques?
    A. They tend to be rough and are not suitable for elderly patients
    B. They are generally well tolerated post surgically
    C. They require active patient participation
    D. The technique is indirect, and therefore the restrictive barrier is not engaged
    E. If the technique fails to work on the first attempt, other techniques should be tried

164. Which is true about rib raising?
    A. It must be performed in inhalation, as the ribs fall in exhalation
    B. An increase of sympathetic activity is typically incurred after an initial decrease
    C. It is a useful technique in patients with viral pneumonia
    D. The technique is autonomic in nature and has little or no effect on chest wall motion
    E. Rib raising must be done in the supine position

165. Which is **FALSE** regarding Spencer techniques?
    A. They are useful in treating adhesive capsulitis
    B. One of the steps requires extension of the arm to 180°
    C. One step requires abduction and internal rotation
    D. Muscle energy techniques can be employed to enhance the Spencer techniques
    E. All of the above are true

166. Stenosis of the intervertebral foramen, resulting in a radiculopathy, which radiates into the upper extremity can be most effectively assessed using which test?
    A. Spurling's test.
    B. Wallenberg's test.
    C. Adson's test.
    D. Roos test.
    E. Speed's test

167. Which one of the following tests will be positive in vertebral artery insufficiency?
    A. Spurling's test.
    B. Wallenberg's test.
    C. Adson's test.
    D. Roos test.
    E. Speed's test.

168. After setting the home run record Mark McGwire comes to your office with left sided shoulder pain. You suspect an overuse injury. In order to evaluate shoulder range of motion you would perform which one of the following tests?
    A. Apley's compression test.
    B. Apley's distraction test.
    C. Apley's scratch test.
    D. Adson's test.
    E. Roos test

169. A positive Adson's test will result from which of the following?
    A. Decreased muscle strength the gluteus medius.
    B. A flexion contracture of the iliopsoas.
    C. Instability of the biceps tendon in the bicipital groove.
    D. Thoracic outlet syndrome.
    E. A rotator cuff tear.

170.. A positive Yergason's test will result from which of the following?
    A. Decreased muscle strength the gluteus medius.
    B. A flexion contracture of the iliopsoas.
    C. Instability of the biceps tendon in the bicipital groove.
    D. Thoracic outlet syndrome.
    E. A rotator cuff tear

171. Which one of the following is true concerning de Quervain's disease?
    A. It results in a flexion contracture of the palmar fascia.
    B. It results from damage to the radial nerve.
    C. It is also known as iliotibial band syndrome.
    D. It results from an inflammation of the abductor pollicis longus and extensor pollicis brevis.
    E. It often results from repetitive and strenuous supination of the forearm.

172. A positive phalen's test in a patient complaining of parasthesia in the upper extremity may lead the practitioner to the diagnosis of:
    A. Thoracic outlet syndrome.
    B. Carpal tunnel syndrome.
    C. A rotator cuff tear.
    D. De Quervain's disease.
    E. Tennis elbow.

173. The hip drop test will be positive in which one of the following conditions?
    A. A group somatic dysfunction in the lumbar spine.
    B. Sciatic nerve root compression.
    C. Neuropathy involving the superior gluteal nerve.
    D. Congenital hip dislocation.
    E. A sacral torsion.

174. The trendelenberg test will assess which one of the following muscle groups.
    A. The hip extensors.
    B. The hip flexors.
    C. The hip abductors.
    D. The hip adductors.
    E. The hip external rotators.

175. A 45 year old male presents to your office with left sided low back pain. He states the pain is worsened by standing up straight after prolonged sitting. The pain radiates to his groin. On examination, you notice that L1 is FR_LS_L, and the he has a tenderpoint medial to his left ASIS. You believe the problem lies within the left hip flexor. Which one of the following tests may aid in confirming your diagnosis?
    A. The hip drop test.
    B. The Thomas test.
    C. Ober's test.
    D. Hoover's test.
    E. The Trendelenberg test.

176. A 32 year old female injured her knee one hour ago playing basketball. As the ER physician, you notice a small joint effusion. She has a positive McMurray's test, and a positive Apley's compression test. Apley's distraction, anterior drawer, and valgus and varus tests are negative. Based on the above information, which one of the following choices is the most likely diagnosis?
    A. chondromalacia patella.
    B. A medial collateral tear.
    C. A lateral collateral tear.
    D. An anterior cruciate tear.
    E. A medial meniscal tear.

177. Excessive anterior movement of the tibia on the femur is indicative of which one of the following conditions?
    A. An ACL injury.
    B. A PCL injury.
    C. A meniscal injury.
    D. A medial collateral injury.
    E. A lateral collateral injury.

178. Which one of the following statements is true concerning Apley's compression test?
    A. Pain elicited with Apley's compression indicates pathology on the posterior surface of the patella.
    B. Apley's compression will be positive in meniscal injuries.
    C. Apley's compression will be positive in ligamentous injuries.
    D. Apley's compression will be positive in both ligamentous and meniscal injuries.
    E. Apley's compression will be positive in rotator cuff tears.

Answer	Page #
1. A	1
2. D	1
3. C	2
4. B	4
5. A	1
6. A	5
7. B	3
8. C	3
9. C	5
10. D	6
11. A	6
12. B	7
13. D	6
14. C	8
15. C	9
16. A	9
17. A	9
18. C	9
19. C	8
20. B	10
21. A	11
22. C	11
23. C	11
24. C	12
25. D	12
26. D	12
27. B	12
28. D	13 & 14
29. D	74
30. A	12
31. B	13
32. C	12
33. B	14
34. C	17
35. C	17 & 18
36. C	16
37. A	16
38. A	19
39. C	18 & 19
40. A	18 & 19
41. D	19
42. B	20
43. B	21
44. D	21

Answer	Page #
45. B	21
46. B	22
47. A	22
48. D	26
49. D	27
50. B	22
51. D	25-27
52. B	25-27
53. C	22
54. C	29
55. B	29
56. D	30
57. E	30
58. E	30
59. C	31
60. B	33
61. D	31
62. A	31
63. D	31
64. C	32
65. B	32
66. B	33
67. C	32
68. B	33
69. E	34
70. B	34
71. C	34
72. D	36
73. B	36
74. D	36
75. A	36
76. C	36
77. E	37
78. D	30
79. D	35 & 36
80. C	38
81. B	38
82. B	40
83. C	40
84. D	42
85. C	41
86. B	40
87. C	41
88. C	42

Answer	Page #
89. C	42
90. B	42
91. B	42
92. B	44
93. A	44
94. D	43
95. B	44
96. B	41
97. A	43
98. D	45
99. D	45 & 46
100.D	46
101.C	47
102.B	47
103.D	47
104.A	48
105.D	48
106.C	50
107.B	50
108.C	50
109.B	50
110.B	50
111.D	50
112.B	50
113.D	52
114.D	56
115.A	51
116.E	51
117.D	51
118.C	51
119.B	51
120.B	58
121.D	57
122.D	53 & 54
123.B	58
124.A	57
125.C	56
126.B	58
127.D	57 & 58
128.C	58
129.A	56
130.A	57
131.B	58
132.D	58

Answer	Page
133.D	57
134.B	56
135.A	57
136.C	57
137.C	58
138.D	56 & 58
139.A	56 & 58
140.C	60
141.B	60
142.C	61
143.C	62
144.E	62 & 63
145.B	63
146.B	63
147.D	64 & 65
148.B	67
149.C	67
150.A	67
151.D	69
152.B	66-68
153.E	69
154.C	70
155.D	71
156.B	71
157.D	72
158.E	74
159.D	71
160.B	78
161.D	79
162.E	79
163.B	86
164.C	86-87
165.B	87
166.A	88
167.B	88
168.C	89
169.D	88
170.C	89
171.D	90
172.B	90
173.A	91
174.C	92
175.B	93
176.E	95

177.A   94
178.B   94

Case A

During the evaluation of a patient's upper back pain, you notice that your right thumb is more posterior upon palpation of the transverse processes of T4. T4 returns to neutral position with extension of the thoracic spine, whereas flexion of the thoracic spine increases the asymmetry.

1. Which of the following is the most correct assessment of T4?
   A. Sidebent left, rotated left
   B. Sidebent right, rotated right
   C. Sidebent right, rotated left
   D. Sidebent left, rotated right
   E. Rotated left, no sidebending component

2. Which of the following is the correct diagnosis?
   A. T4 NS_LR_R
   B. T4 FR_LS_L
   C. T4 ER_RS_R
   D. T4 NS_RR_L
   E. T4 ER_LS_L

3. Which of the following organs would be **LEAST** affected by an autonomic imbalance at T4?
   A. Heart
   B. Esophagus
   C. Stomach
   D. Lungs
   E. Tongue

4. If treating this patient with HVLA from a supine position, which of the following is **CORRECT** regarding hand placement and direction of force?
   A. The thenar eminence is placed under the right transverse process of T5, force is perpendicular to the table
   B. The thenar eminence is placed under the right transverse process of T4, force is perpendicular to the table
   C. The thenar eminence is placed under the right transverse process of T3, force is 45° caudad
   D. The thenar eminence is placed under the right transverse process of T4, force is 45° cephalad
   E. The thenar eminence is placed under the right transverse process of T5, force is 45° cephalad

Case B

A 30 year old athletic male presents to your office complaining of low back pain. He states that the pain started soon after playing baseball. The pain is localized to his low back. He denies any radiation of pain, parasthesias or weakness in the lower extremities, "saddle anesthesia" or incontinence. There is no previous history of low back pain. Physical exam reveals no focal neurologic deficits. X-rays of the lumbar spine are normal. There is marked spasm of the paraspinal musculature on the right. There appears to be a group dysfunction from L1-L5 that is markedly rotated right and sidebent left.

5. Which of the following is the most likely diagnosis?
    A. Lumbar spinal stenosis
    B. Sciatica
    C. Acute lumbar strain
    D. Herniated nucleus pulposus
    E. Spondylolisthesis

6. If the patient had reported decreased sensation on the medial aspect of the ankle, absent patellar reflex and marked weakness of ankle dorsiflexion and knee extension, what would the most likely diagnosis be?
    A. Spondylolisthesis
    B. Lumbar spinal stenosis
    C. Herniated nucleus pulposus
    D. Acute lumbar strain
    E. None of the above are likely diagnoses

7. If there is a somatic dysfunction at the sacrum that is associated with the L5 dysfunction, which would be expected?
    A. Left rotation on Right oblique axis
    B. Right rotation on Left oblique axis
    C. Left rotation on Left oblique axis
    D. Right rotation on Right oblique axis
    E. Right margin posterior

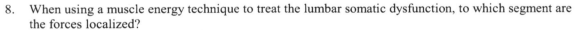

8. When using a muscle energy technique to treat the lumbar somatic dysfunction, to which segment are the forces localized?
    A. L1
    B. L2
    C. L3
    D. L4
    E. L5

9. The patient is found to have a tenderpoint 1cm lateral to the pubic symphysis on the superior pubic ramus. This tenderpoint correlates to somatic dysfunction of which vertebra?
    A. L1
    B. L2
    C. L3
    D. L4
    E. L5

10. Which of the following is the correct treatment position for the above tenderpoint?
    A. Patient prone, knees flexed, hips extended, rotated to contralateral side
    B. Patient prone, knees flexed, hips extended, rotated to ipsilateral side
    C. Patient supine, knees flexed, hips extended, rotated to contralateral side
    D. Patient supine, knees and hips flexed, rotated to ipsilateral side
    E. Patient supine, knees and hips flexed, rotated to contralateral side

Case C

A 25 year old graduate student comes into your office complaining of left-sided neck pain radiating to the shoulder. The pain began a few days after finals' week, during which the patient spent nearly 100 hours working at his desk. The cardiac workup, including EKG, demonstrates no abnormality. Deep tendon reflexes are normal, and Adson's test is negative. During your structural examination, you locate a tenderpoint in the posterior scalene muscle. You also note that translation of the OA is induced more easily to the right and becomes more symmetrical in flexion. C5 translates more easily to the left and becomes more symmetrical in extension.

11. Which of the following is the correct diagnosis of the somatic dysfunction at C5?
    A. C5 FR_LS_R
    B. C5 FR_LS_L
    C. C5 FR_RS_L
    D. C5 ER_RS_R
    E. C5 ER_LS_L

12. Which of the following describe the restriction at the OA?
    A. Extension, right sidebending, left rotation
    B. Extension, right sidebending, right rotation
    C. Extension, left sidebending, right rotation
    D. Flexion, left sidebending, right rotation
    E. Flexion, right sidebending, left rotation

13. A tenderpoint in the posterior scalene muscle is commonly associated with which rib dysfunction?
    A. 1st Rib inhalation dysfunction
    B. 2nd Rib inhalation dysfunction
    C. 1st Rib exhalation dysfunction
    D. 3rd-5th Ribs inhalation dysfunction
    E. 3rd-5th Ribs exhalation dysfunction

14. Which of the following is true regarding the neck pain of this patient?
    A. It is best treated with HVLA since acute dysfunctions respond best to quick treatment
    B. It is best treated with indirect techniques to avoid further strain
    C. It is best to treat the shoulder before addressing the cervical region
    D. It is important to treat the cervical spine before addressing the upper thoracic region
    E. It is best to order x-rays of the cervical spine before attempting any manipulation

15. In order to properly perform Adson's test, which of the following must occur?
    A. The patient turns their head to the contralateral side
    B. Flexion of the elbow
    C. Palpation of the radial pulse
    D. Internal rotation of the shoulder
    E. The arm must be freely allowed to drop

16. Which of the following organs are **NOT** affected by an autonomic imbalance at the OA?
    A. Liver
    B. Gallbladder
    C. Heart
    D. Urinary bladder
    E. Both A and B are correct

127

Case D

A 34 year old female comes into your office complaining of mild left-sided thoracic pain. The pain started about a week after the patient began driving her new sports car which has very low riding seats. The pain is non-radiating and worsens with inhalation. X-rays and EKG reveal no abnormalities. Your structural exam reveals that ribs 3-5 on the left are more caudad and lag behind during inhalation. Tenderpoints are noted on ribs 3-5 in the left mid axillary line.

17. Which of the following is the correct dysfunction?
    A. Left rib 3-5 inhalation dysfunction
    B. Left rib 3-5 exhalation dysfunction
    C. Right rib 3-5 inhalation dysfunction
    D. Right rib 3-5 exhalation dysfunction

18. At which rib is treatment directed?
    A. Rib 2
    B. Rib 3
    C. Rib 4
    D. Rib 5
    E. Rib 6

19. If a muscle energy technique is used to treat this dysfunction, will muscle will be used?
    A. Anterior and Middle scalene
    B. Posterior scalene
    C. Pectoralis minor
    D. Serratus anterior
    E. Latissimus dorsi

20. If a group thoracic dysfunction from T3-T5 is associated with the rib dysfunction, to which of the following vertebra is treatment directed?
    A. T2
    B. T3
    C. T4
    D. T5
    E. T6

Questions 21 and 22 are not related to the above case

21. Which of the following statements concerning treatment of rib dysfunction is true?
    A. Thoracic dysfunctions should be treated before rib dysfunctions
    B. Exhalation dysfunctions cannot be treated with HVLA
    C. The tenderpoints are treated by rotating and sidebending the thorax away from the dysfunction
    D. Muscle energy techniques are contraindicated in elderly patients with COPD
    E. An inhalation dysfunction of ribs 6-9 can be corrected by contracting the serratus anterior muscle.

22. Which of the following tenderpoint locations are associated with inhalation rib dysfunctions?
    A. Mid axillary line
    B. Mid clavicular line
    C. Articulation of the rib and sternum
    D. Angle of the rib
    E. Costochondral articulation

Case E

A 53 year old male patient presents complaining of low back pain of recent onset. You are able to rule out genitourinary and gastrointestinal etiologies of his pain. There are also no palpable abdominal masses. You suspect a neuro-musculoskeletal etiology of the pain.

23. An MRI on this patient reveals a posteriolateral disc herniation at the L5-S-1 disc space. Which of the following tests would you expect to be positive?
    - A. Straight leg raising test
    - B. Thomas Test
    - C. Hip drop test
    - D. Ober's test
    - E. Phalen's test

24. Which of the following physical signs may be observed in the above patient if there was compression of the S1 nerve root?
    - A. Decreased ability for the patient to walk on his toes
    - B. Decreased ability for the patient to walk on his heels
    - C. 0/4 patellar tendon reflex
    - D. Decreased sensation on the dorsum of the foot
    - E. Sustained clonus with ankle dorsiflexion

25. Which of the following symptoms would be strongly suggestive of "cauda equina" syndrome in the above patient?
    - A. Radiation of pain to legs
    - B. Loss of sensation on the lateral thigh
    - C. Palpable pulsating mass
    - D. 2/4 deep tendon reflexes in the lower extremity
    - E. Urinary incontinence

26. Which of the following terms and definitions are correctly matched?
    - A. Spondylolisthesis ↔ Degenerative disc changes
    - B. Spondylolysis ↔ Narrowing of intervertebral foramina
    - C. Spondylosis ↔ Fracture of pars interarticularis
    - D. Spondylolysis ↔ No anterior displacement of the vertebral body
    - E. Spondylolisthesis ↔ Ankylosing of adjacent vertebral bodies

27. Which of the following organs would be **least** affected by an autonomic imbalance of the upper lumbar spine?
    - A. Ureters
    - B. Urinary bladder
    - C. Transverse colon
    - D. Penis
    - E. Adrenal medulla

Case F

A 34 year old female enters your office complaining of hip pain following a fall off of a stepladder. X-rays taken in the emergency room revealed no fracture, and the patient has been very uncomfortable for the past four days. The pain is localized on the left, and <u>does not</u> radiate down the thigh. The left ASIS is cephalad and the left PSIS is caudad. While performing a standing flexion test, you note that the left PSIS demonstrated greater excursion than the right.

28. Which of the following would you expect to find in this patient?
    A. Restricted AP compression on the right
    B. Left iliosacral dysfunction
    C. Longer leg on the left
    D. L5 $NS_L R_R$
    E. Exquisite pain upon palpation of the pubic symphysis

29. What is the pelvic diagnosis?
    A. Left innominate anterior
    B. Left innominate posterior
    C. Right innominate anterior
    D. Right innominate posterior
    E. Not enough information to determine

30. Which of the following soft tissue dysfunctions is <u>most likely</u> to cause this pelvic dysfunction?
    A. Tight quadriceps
    B. Tight hip adductors
    C. Tight hip abductors
    D. Tight hamstrings
    E. Tight piriformis

31. If this patient presented with a positive Thomas test on the right, which lumbar somatic dysfunction would you expect to find?
    A. L1 $NS_L R_R$
    B. L2 $ES_L R_R$
    C. L3 $NS_L R_R$
    D. L1 $FR_R S_R$
    E. L4 $FS_L R_R$

32. Which of the following statements about the muscle energy treatment of this pelvic dysfunction is true?
    A. Hip flexors are used to correct the dysfunction
    B. The patient must be treated from the seated position
    C. The patient's hip is flexed and slightly abducted
    D. Hip extensors are activated by the patient to correct the dysfunction
    E. Muscle energy treatment is relatively contraindicated in the above patient

Case G

A 53 year old obese male with a 10 year history of Type II diabetes mellitus presents to your office complaining of low back pain radiating to the right buttocks. The pain started 3-4 weeks ago and has gradually increased. The PSIS's are equal and the lumbosacral spring test is positive. The right sulcus is deeper, and the right ILA is deeper. The left sulcus is the only corner of the sacrum that resists springing. An anterior lumbar tenderpoint is found on the right. Patellar and Achilles reflexes are 1/4 bilaterally with no gross sensory deficits. Muscle testing is 4+/5 throughout. X-rays reveal no abnormalities.

33. Which of the following would you definitively expect to find in this patient?
    A. Somatic dysfunction of the lower extremities
    B. Positive standing flexion test on the right
    C. Lumbar curve convex to the right
    D. Positive seated flexion test on the left
    E. Reduced asymmetry of the sulci with lumbar extension

34. Which of the following is the correct sacral diagnosis?
    A. Left rotation on Right oblique axis
    B. Right rotation on Left oblique axis
    C. Left unilateral sacral flexion
    D. Right unilateral sacral extension
    E. Right margin posterior

35. Which of the following L5 findings is associated with the above dysfunction?
    A. NS_RR_L
    B. NS_LR_R
    C. FR_RS_R
    D. FR_LS_L
    E. There is no L5 dysfunction associated with the above sacral dysfunction

36. Which of the following soft tissue dysfunctions is most likely to be associated with the above sacral dysfunction?
    A. Contracture spasm of the rectus abdominus
    B. Positive Ober's test
    C. Piriformis tenderpoint
    D. Lumbar intervertebral disc degeneration
    E. Quadratus lumborum tenderpoint

37. Which of the following is true regarding the above patient?
    A. Treatment should be directed at L5 first
    B. The L5 dysfunction can be treated using muscle energy with the patient in the left lateral Sim's position
    C. HVLA is absolutely contraindicated in this patient due to the likelihood of disc herniation
    D. The lumbar tenderpoint is treated with the hips extended
    E. Due to the presence of type II diabetes mellitus and the decreased deep tendon reflexes, muscle energy is absolutely contraindicated

38. Which of the following is **FALSE** regarding the disposition of the patient after this office visit?
    A. Hemoglobin A1c should be monitored
    B. The patient should receive a comprehensive eye examination every six months
    C. Lipid levels should be monitored
    D. An MRI to assess the lumbar discs should be performed
    E. The patient should be given advice regarding weight loss and exercise

Case H

A 72 year old male comes to your office complaining of new onset right shoulder pain. The pain started two days ago during his golf tournament. The patient recalls that the pain came about immediately following a golf swing. The pain, which is greatest at the tip of the right acromion, does not radiate. He denies and numbness or tingling in his upper extremity. There is full passive range of motion, but the pain worsens with any active movement of the arm.

39. You instruct your patient to abduct his arms and then slowly lower them. When he attempts to comply, you notice that he is unable to slowly lower the right arm for the first half of the way down. What disorder does this suggest?
    A. Adhesive capsulitis
    B. Bicipital tendinitis
    C. Osteoarthrosis of the glenohumeral joint
    D. Rotator cuff tear
    E. Thoracic outlet syndrome

40. The above patient has a history of hemophilia A, which of the following would you be most concerned about?
    A. Early arthritic degeneration of the synovium
    B. Gout-like crystalline synovium
    C. Collagen/vascular disease predisposing to grade 3 sprain
    D. Hemarthrosis
    E. Rhabdomyolysis

41. Given the patient's history and physical findings, which of the following is **NOT** indicated?
    A. Heat
    B. Rest
    C. Ice
    D. Fascial release of the shoulder
    E. Acetaminophen

42. If the above patient has a neurological deficit resulting in an absent triceps tendon reflex is on the right, a loss of sensation on the dorsum of the hand, and weakness in the the extensors of the hand, wrist and elbow. Which nerve is most likely involved?
    A. Musculocutaneous
    B. Median
    C. Radial
    D. Ulnar
    E. Axillary

Case I

You are assessing a 2 month old infant. The child was delivered at 40 weeks by spontaneous vaginal delivery complicated by shoulder dystocia. At birth the child was 10lbs 2oz. in weight and measured 35 cm head to toe. The Apgars were 9 and 10. You note that the OA is visibly sidebent left and there is a positive Ortolani sign.

43. Which of the following is most likely to be associated with a positive Ortolani sign?
    A. Ambylopia
    B. Klumpke's palsy
    C. Erb-Duchenne's palsy
    D. Bell's palsy
    E. Congenital dislocation of the hip

44. Which of the following is most commonly associated with Erb-Duchenne's palsy?
    A. +3/4 biceps tendon reflex on the ipsilateral side
    B. Decreased radial pulse
    C. Inability to supinate
    D. Inability to smile or frown on ipsilateral side
    E. C7 somatic dysfunction

45. If the above patient was diagnosed with Erb's palsy, which of the following treatments would never be used in this patient?
    A. Cranial manipulation
    B. Myofascial release
    C. Articulatory techniques
    D. Direct techniques
    E. Muscle energy techniques

46. What is the most likely cause of the shoulder dystocia?
    A. The child was delivered preterm
    B. The child was macrosomic
    C. The mother did not receive prenatal care
    D. The physician probably used forceps during delivery
    E. The child was not apparently healthy at delivery

Case J

You are examining a 61 year old male patient with new onset CHF. He is on his second hospital day, and serial chest x-rays demonstrate a decreasing quantity of pulmonary vascular congestion in both lung fields. The patient states that he has had large bouts of indigestion for the past week, after which a nonproductive incessant cough began two day prior to admission. The EKG taken in the emergency department demonstrated 4 mm Q-waves in leads II, III and aVF. The CK-MB is elevated, but declining over the past 24 hours. Albumin, PT and PTT are all normal.

47. Which of the following is the etiology of the CHF?
    A. Gastritis with secondary portal hypertension
    B. Liver failure secondary to portal hypertension
    C. Pneumonia leading to cor pulmonale
    D. Myocardial infarction of the inferior wall
    E. Pulmonary embolus complicated by cor pulmonale

48. Which of the following would you **NOT** expect to find in this patient as a result of the above signs and symptoms?
    A. T3-T5 $NS_L R_R$
    B. Right rib 3-5 inhalation dysfunction
    C. Right pectoralis minor tenderpoint
    D. L5 $ER_L S_L$
    E. T2 $FR_R S_R$

49. Which of the following is FALSE about myocardial infarction?
    A. It can cause a fatal arrhythmia resulting in sudden cardiac death
    B. It can lead to CHF
    C. Patients can present with jaw or left shoulder pain
    D. Diabetics are acutely sensitive to early signs of ischemia
    E. Myocardial infarction rarely leads to somatic dysfunction

50. Which of the following techniques would **MOST** improve this patient's CHF?
    A. Thoracic lymph pump to increase lymphatic return.
    B. Counterstrain to any tenderpoints that are caused by a viscero-somatic reflex
    C. Redome the diaphragm to improve respiratory dysfunction.
    D. HVLA to restore symmetry in the thoracic spine.
    E. Rib raising to normalize parasympathetic tone.

Case K

You are examining a 29 year old male presenting to the emergency room complaining of right sided flank pain. The pain is intermittent, excruciating and radiates to the right testicle. There is no rebound tenderness or signs of peritoneal irritation. There is costovertebral angle tenderness on the right. The patient is afebrile, mildly hypertensive, tachycardic and diaphoretic. The urinalysis demonstrates RBCs too numerous to count, small leukocytes and negative for nitrites. The CBC is normal. KUB demonstrates a 6 mm well circumscribed radio-opaque mass approximately 10 cm superior to the middle of the right pubic ramus. IVP confirms the presence and location of the stone with severe hydronephrosis.

51. Which of the following would be the appropriate course of action?
    A. Limit fluid intake.
    B. Discharge the patient home to follow up with their primary care physician within 48 hours.
    C. Call to schedule an emergency appendectomy to remove the fecalith
    D. Order a urology consult
    E. Order a CT of the pelvis

52. Which of the following soft tissue dysfunctions is likely to be caused as a result of the patients diagnosis?
    A. Right psoas tenderpoint
    B. Abdominal rectus spasm
    C. Piriformis tenderpoint
    D. T10-L2 somatic dysfunction
    E. Left inferior pubic shear

53. Which of the following is likely to be associated with the above dysfunction?
    A. Lumbar somatic dysfunction
    B. Right superior pubic shear
    C. Unilateral sacral dysfunction
    D. Positive seated flexion test on the left
    E. Positive straight leg raising test

54. What is the most likely composition of the mass in the KUB?
    A. Struvite
    B. Uric acid
    C. Calcium oxalate
    D. Cystine
    E. Bile pigment

Case L

You are examining a 32 year old secretary who complains of numbness and tingling in both hands. The symptoms are isolated to the palmar surface of the thumb, index and middle fingers. The symptoms are worse at night. On examination, there is no atrophy or weakness noted at the thenar eminences. There are no radiographic abnormalities and deep tendon reflexes are 2/4 bilaterally.

55. Which of the following tests is considered the gold standard for diagnosis of carpal tunnel syndrome?

    A. Bone scan
    B. Thermography
    C. Finkelstein's test
    D. Tinel's, Phalen's and Prayer tests
    E. Nerve conduction and electromyographic studies

56. Which treatment should be done first when using OMT to treat this patient?

    A. Myofascial release of the flexor retinaculum
    B. Myofascial release of the palmar surface
    C. Muscle energy / counterstrain to the forearm musculature
    D. Correction of somatic dysfunction in the carpal bones
    E. Correction of cervical somatic dysfunction

57. A symptom associated with an increased pressure in the carpal tunnel is:
    A. Weakness in abduction and adduction of the fingers.
    B. Loss of sensation of the little finger
    C. Decreased muscle strength in opposition of the thumb
    D. A positive Adson's test.
    E. Loss of sensation on the dorsum of the hand.

58. When addressing sympathetic tone in the arm, which is the most important area to consider?
    A. C5-C7
    B. OA
    C. T5-T7
    D. The clavicle, due to its proximity to the brachial plexus
    E. The sacrum

Case M

You are examining a 22 year old female with a history of temporomandibular disorder. She often experiences "pain and popping" of her right temporomandibular joint while eating. When the pain is severe, it usually results in a headache. On examination, you notice crepitus and left deviation of the jaw on opening.

59. Which of the following would not be considered a first line treatment for this patient?
    - A. Heat
    - B. OMT
    - C. Craniosacral therapy
    - D. NSAIDs
    - E. Muscle relaxants

60. Which of the following is **FALSE** regarding behavior modification for treatment of this patient?
    - A. The patient should be instructed to do stretches for the muscles of mastication regularly.
    - B. The patient may wear a bite plate while sleeping.
    - C. The patient should exercise her jaw by eating chewy foods, like gum or taffy.
    - D. The patient should utilize ice alternately with heat at the preauricular region.
    - E. All of the above are true.

61. If this patient were also presenting with tinnitus, which cranial nerve would you expect to be involved?
    - A. II
    - B. IV
    - C. VII
    - D. VIII
    - E. XI

62. Which of the following is **FALSE** regarding the temporomandibular joint?
    - A. It is the articulation of the temporal bone and the condylar process of the mandible
    - B. It is a synovial joint
    - C. TMJ symptoms are present in less then 1% of the U.S. population
    - D. The joint contains an articular disc
    - E. It is anatomically close to the mandibular nerve

Case N

A 13 year old male presents to your office with right wrist and elbow pain following a fall on his outstretched arm. On examination, there is no edema or ecchymosis around the wrist or elbow. Passive supination of the forearm is decreased on the right. There is tenderness in the anatomic snuffbox and a tenderpoint at the musculotendinous insertion of the lateral epicondyle. X-rays of the wrist and elbow are normal.

63. Based on the history and physical findings, what is the most likely diagnosis?
    A. Adducted ulna
    B. Posterior radial head
    C. Abducted ulna
    D. Carpal tunnel syndrome
    E. Medial epicondylitis

64. All of the following are valid treatments for this dysfunction **EXCEPT**:
    A. Muscle energy to the upper extremity to increase supination
    B. Counterstrain to the tenderpoint
    C. NSAIDs to decrease local inflammation
    D. HVLA to the wrist to improve range of motion
    E. Myofascial release to decease restrictions

65. The patient returns one week later with moderate inflammation around the wrist. The pain has worsened significantly in that time. Which of the following would be the appropriate course of action?
    A. Prescribe a more effective pain medication have the child follow up in a week
    B. Repeat the x-ray of the wrist, even though the first set was normal, then immobilize the wrist for three months
    C. Immobilize the wrist for 2 weeks with a cast
    D. Reassure the parent and the child that the inflammation and pain is typical of wrist sprains
    E. None of the above are correct

Case A

1. **B** **Sidebent right rotated right**. If your right thumb is posterior, this indicates right rotation. Extending returns T4 to the neutral position indicating an extended type II somatic dysfunction. Fryette's principles states that in a non-neutral (extended in this case) dysfunction sidebending and rotation are to the same side. If it's rotated right, then it must be sidebent right.

2. **C** **T4 ER_RS_R**. If T4 returns to the neutral position when the spine is extended, then T4 must be extended (name it for the way it wants to go).

3. **C** **Stomach**. The stomach receives autonomic innervation from T5-T9. All other answers receive a portion of their autonomic innervation from T4 (Heart T1-T5, Esophagus T2-T8, Lungs T2-T7, Head and Neck T1-T4.

4. **E** **The thenar eminence is placed under the right transverse process of T5, force is directed 45^0 cephalad**. Using the Kirksville Krunch technique, to reverse all planes of a T4 ER_RS_R the physician's thenar eminence is placed under the right transverse process of T5 (to induce left rotation of the spine and extension of T5, thus flexion of T4). The trust in then 45^0 cephalad. See page 82 for procedure.

Case B

5. **C** **Acute Lumbar Strain**. An acute lumbar strain is low back pain without focal neurological deficits. The pain may be sharp or dull, and usually localized to the low back, although it may radiate in a nondermatomal type of fashion. Spinal stenosis is a chronic joint disease characterized by slowly developing joint pain, usually resulting from intervertebral narrowing, foraminal encroachment and / or spinal canal compression. Sciatica is typically low buttock pain with radiation of pain into the thigh or leg. Sciatica may accompany low back pain and may be caused by a herniated disc or osteoarthosis [7 p.187] A herniated nucleus pulposus (herniated disc) will often result in neurologic deficits therefore making this an unlikely diagnosis. Spondylolisthesis is a forward slippage of the lumbar vertebrae. Radiographic findings in this case are normal making this an unlikely diagnosis.

6. **C** **Herniated nucleus pulposus**. A herniated disc will result in decreased sensation, decreased deep tendon reflexes and lower extremity weakness. Radiographic findings on the patent was normal making spondylolisthesis unlikely. Spinal stenosis is usually due to intervertebral narrowing and degenerative joint disease. Also, lumbar spinal stenosis is usually seen in the middle age or elderly population.

7. **C** **Left rotation on a Left oblique axis**. L5 will influence the sacrum in the following ways: if L5 is rotated the sacrum will rotate in the opposite way on an oblique axis. If L5 is sidebent, the sacral oblique is engaged on the same side. Since the patient's L5 was NSLRR, the sacrum must be rotated left on a left oblique axis.

8. **C** **L3**. When treating a group somatic dysfunction of the axial skeleton, forces should be directed to the apex of the curve. In this case L3.

9. **E** **L5**. Anterior lumbar tenderpoints are located about the pelvis. L5 is located approximately 1 cm lateral to the pubic symphysis on the superior rami. L2 to L4 are located at the AIIS. L1 is located a the ASIS.

10. **E** **Patent supine, knees and hips flexed, rotated to the contralateral side**. Most anterior lumbar tenderpoints are treated in the above fashion (see page 68 for further details).

Case C

11. **D c5 ER$_R$S$_R$.** Since C5 translates more easily to the left it must be sidebent to the right. Remember that C2-C7 sidebend and rotate to the same side, therefore C5 must be rotated right. Since C5 translates symmetrically in extension it must be extended.

12. **A Extension right sidebending, left rotation.** Since the OA translates more easily to the right it must be sidebent left (and restricted in right sidebending). Remember, the OA rotates and sidebends to opposite sides, therefore it must be rotated right (and restricted in left rotation). Since the OA translates symmetrically in flexion it must be flexed (and restricted in extension).

13. **B 2nd rib inhalation dysfunction.** The posterior scalene originates from the transverse process of C4 - C6 and inserts onto the second rib. Tenderness of this muscle is most commonly associated with a rib 2 dysfunction. Tenderness in the anterior scalene may be associated with a rib 1 dysfunction. Tenderness in the pectoralis minor may be associated with dysfunctions of ribs 3-5.

14. **B It is best to treat with indirect techniques to avoid further strain.** With indirect techniques, the tissue is taken away from the restrictive barrier and usually allowed to relax. These techniques are gentle and are tolerated well in acute situations. Acute neck strains may actually worsen with HVLA techniques. It is best to treat the axial skeleton before treating shoulder or extremity problems. For acute somatic dysfunctions treat the secondary or peripheral areas to allow access to the acute area. Based on the age, history and physical findings, X-rays are not indicated in this patient especially if indirect treatment is attempted.

15. **C Palpation of the radial pulse.** Adson's test is for thoracic outlet syndrome and assessment of the subclavian artery. For a full description on how to perform the test see Chapter 16 Special Tests section II A on page 88.

16. **D Urinary Bladder.** Somatic dysfunction of the OA will effect the vagus nerve (page 50). The vagus nerve has parasympathetic control of the thoracic and upper abdominal viscera. The pelvic splanchnic nerve controls the parasympathetic functions of the urinary bladder.

Case D

17. **B Left rib 3-5 Exhalation dysfunction.** Exhalation dysfunctions are characterized by one or a group of ribs stuck down. These ribs typically lag behind in inhalation. Pain usually increases with inhalation. Also anterior rib tenderpoints (in the mid axillary line) are often associated with anteriorly depressed ribs.

18. **B Rib 3** In a group dysfunction usually one "key" rib is responsible in causing the dysfunction. In exhalation dysfunctions the "key" rib is the uppermost rib of the dysfunction.

19. **C Pectoralis minor.** As above ribs 3-5 are stuck in exhalation. The pectoralis minor muscle originates from the coracoid process and inserts on ribs 3-5. Activation of this muscle with muscle energy would pull the shaft of the ribs superior, correcting the dysfunction.

20. **C T4.** When treating a group somatic dysfunction of the axial skeleton, forces should be directed to the apex of the curve. In this case T4.

21. **A** **Thoracic dysfunctions should be treated before rib dysfunctions**. Rib dysfunctions may be caused by corresponding thoracic dysfunctions. If a thoracic dysfunction is present treat the thoracic spine before treating the specific rib dysfunction. Rib exhalation dysfunctions can be treated using the Kirksville Krunch technique (see page 83). Anterior rib tenderpoints are treated by rotating and sidebending the thorax *toward* the dysfunction. Although muscle energy techniques should not be performed on patients with low vitality who could be compromised by adding muscular exertion, elderly patients with COPD can typically manage active muscular contraction without exacerbating their COPD. An *exhalation* dysfunction of ribs 6-9 can be corrected with muscle energy by contracting the serratus anterior.

22. **D** Posterior tenderpoints are associated with posteriorly depressed ribs (inhalation dysfunctions). Posterior rib tenderpoints are located on the angle of the corresponding rib.

Case E

23. **A** **Straight leg raising test**. The straight leg raising test is used to evaluate the lumbar spine and sciatic nerve compression. A patient with herniated disc will experience pain when the lower extremity is passively raised. Other answers are as follows: Thomas test - flexion contracture of the iliopsoas, Hip drop test - asymmetrical lumbar sidebending, Ober's test - tight iliotibial band, Phalen's test - carpal tunnel syndrome.

24. **A** **Decreased ability of the patient to walk on their toes**. Although the S1 nerve root innervates several parts of the lower extremity, it is intimately involved in plantar flexion of the foot. Decreased ability to walk on his heels and 0/4 patella reflex may indicate pathology of the L4 nerve root. Sensation at the dorsum of the foot is supplied by L5. Sustained ankle clonus is associated with an upper motor neuron lesion; a herniated disc at L5-S1 would result in nerve root (lower motor neuron) compression.

25. **E** **Urinary incontinence**. Cauda equina syndrome may result in saddle anesthesia, decreased deep tendon reflexes, decreased rectal tone and loss of bowel and bladder control. Although the patient may complain of pain radiating into the lower extremities, this symptom may also be caused by other low back pathology such as a herniated disc or spinal stenosis.

26. **D** **Spondylolysis ↔ No anterior displacement of the vertebral body**. Spondylolysis results from a fracture in the pars interarticularis without anterior displacement of the vertebral body. It is usually seen as a collar on the scotty dog on lumbar X-rays. Other answers are as follows: Spondylosis ↔Degenerative disc changes and ankylosing of adjacent vertebral bodies, Spondylolisthesis ↔ Anterior displacement of one vertebrae on another.

27. **E** **Adrenal medulla**. The adrenal medulla receives sympathetic innervation from T10. Other answers are as follows: ureters T10-L2, urinary bladder T11-L2, transverse colon T10-L2, Penis T11-L2.

Case F

28. **B** **Left iliosacral dysfunction**. The case describes a positive standing flexion test on the left. The standing flexion test evaluates iliosacral dysfunction, therefore a positive standing flexion test on the left would indicate a left iliosacral dysfunction.

29. **B** **Left innominate posterior**. A positive standing flexion test on the left indicates a left innominate problem. The left ASIS is cephalad and the left PSIS is caudad, these findings are indicative of posterior innominate on the left.

30. **D** **Tight hamstrings**. The most common etiology of a left innominate posterior is tight hamstrings.

31. **D L1 FR$_R$S$_R$**. A positive Thomas test is indicative of a flexion contracture of the iliopsoas. This is often associated with a non-neutral dysfunction of L1 or L2.

32. **A Hip flexors are used to correct the dysfunction**. The treatment position to correct a left innominate posterior is as follows. With the patient supine, drop the left leg off the table to engage the restrictive barrier. Instruct the patient to flex their hip against your counterforce for 3-5 seconds.

Case G

33. **D Positive seated flexion test on the left**. The patient in the above case has a sacral somatic dysfunction. The sacrum has rotated left on a right oblique axis. This will result in a positive seated flexion test on the left (seated flexion test positive on the opposite side of the axis). Somatic dysfunction of the lower extremities may or may not accompany a sacral torsion. A positive standing flexion test will result from an innominate dysfunction, not a sacral torsion. A left on right sacral torsion will result in a lumbar curve that is convex to the *left*. Selection E is describing a negative backward bending test; in a L on R torsion, the backward bending would be positive.

34. **A Left rotation on a right oblique axis**. Since the lumbosacral spring test is positive, part or all of the sacral base has moved posterior. The sacral sulcus on the right is deeper, therefore the left is more shallow and must have moved posterior. The right ILA is deeper, making the only possible diagnosis a L on R. A R on L, right margin posterior and a right USE would all produce a shallow right sulcus. A left USF will produce a deep left sulcus and a negative lumbosacral spring.

35. **C FR$_R$S$_R$**. Following the rules of L5 on the sacrum: The sacrum is rotated left therefore L5 is rotated right. The sacrum has a right oblique axis, therefore L5 is sidebent right. Following Fryette's principle II, if sidebending and rotation are to the same side, then L5 must be non-neutral (flexed or extended).

36. **C Piriformis tenderpoint**. Piriformis tenderpoints are often associated with sacral dysfunctions. [25 p.235] Spasm of the rectus abdominus is associated with superior pubic shear. A positive Ober's test is associated with a tight iliotibial band. Although the above patient may have lumbar disk degeneration or a quadratus lumborum tenderpoint, these findings are not associated with a sacral dysfunction.

37. **A Treatment should be directed toward L5 first**. Sacral dysfunctions will often spontaneously resolve with treatment of L5 (p.28). The *sacral torsion* can be treated using muscle energy with the patient in the right lateral Sim's position. Anterior lumbar tenderpoints are typically treated with the hips flexed. The above patient is unlikely to have a disc herniation, because the onset of pain is gradual and the decreased reflexes are most likely due to diabetic neuropathy. Therefore, HVLA would not be contraindicated. Muscle energy is only contraindicated in patient's with low vitality, such as ICU patients and post-surgical patients.

38. **D An MRI to assess the lumbar discs should be performed**. Conservative therapy and lumbar x-rays are indicated to rule out more common causes of low back pain such as degenerative joint disease. All diabetics should have their HgA1c and lipid levels monitored. They should also receive a comprehensive eye exam every six months to check for retinopathy and all should be given advise regarding weight loss and exercise.

Case H

39. **D Rotator cuff tear**. The question describes a positive drop arm test. A rotator cuff tear is often associated with trauma and will result in sharp at the tip of the acromion, weakness in active abduction and a positive drop arm test. Restricted range of motion is characteristic of adhesive capsulitis. Bicipital tendinitis will result in pain at the bicipital grove and increased pain with supination and flexion and extension at the elbow. Osteoarthrosis is characterized by a gradual onset of pain and limited passive range of motion. Thoracic outlet syndrome is due to compression of the neurovascular bundle. This typically results in pain radiating into the upper extremity.

40. **D Hemarthrosis**. Hemophiliacs are at great risk of bleeding, even from minor trauma. Hemarthrosis (blood in a joint) must be considered especially of the patient has increased joint edema and a gradual decreasing range of motion.

41. **A Heat**. Initial therapy for a musculoskeletal injury would include rest and ice. Heat may be attempted 48 hours post-injury. A fascial release of the shoulder may be attempted to decreased myofascial restrictions and improve lymphatic return to reduce edema and promote healing. Aspirin and NSAIDS are not suggested for analgesia in hemophiliacs due to the increased risk of bleeding. For these patients acetaminophen is suggested.

42. **C Radial**. The radial nerve innervates the extensors of the upper extremity (elbow wrist and hand). Sensation to the first three digits on the dorsum of the hand is supplied by the radial nerve. The triceps are innervated by the radial nerve, therefore a absent reflex will indicate radial nerve pathology.

Case I

43. **E Congenital dislocation of the hip**. Ortolani's test can be used to diagnose congenital hip dislocation. It is performed by flexing and abducting the hips while exerting pressure on the greater trochanters. It is positive of the physician feels a "clunk" which indicates that the hip joint has been reduced. [6 p. 347-8]

44. **C Inability to supinate**. Erb's palsy is an upper arm paralysis caused by injury to the C5 and C6 nerve roots. It can result in paralysis of the deltoid, external rotators, biceps, brachioradialis and supinator muscles.

45. **E Muscle energy techniques**. Muscle energy is an active treatment and requires isometric activation of various muscles. If the patient had Erb's palsy, he would never be able to actively contract some of the muscles in his arm. All other techniques listed may be done passively and does not require patient participation.

46. **B The child was macrosomic**. Shoulder dystocia is often associated with macrosomia. Any neonate weighing over 4000g is considered macrosomic. Post-term deliveries and gestational diabetes are common causes of macrosomia.

Case J

47. **D Myocardial infarction of the inferior wall**. CHF can often occur as a result of an MI. Other common causes include hypertension and valvular disease. Q waves in leads II, III, and aVF are characteristic of an inferior MI. Gastritis, liver failure, pneumonia and pulmonary embolism are all unlikely diagnoses considering this patient's symptoms.

48. **D L5 ER$_L$S$_L$**. The heart receives autonomic innervation from T1-T5, therefore any abnormal sensory input from the heart can alter the output and cause somatic dysfunction of T1-T5. The above patient also had a cough. A persistent cough can alter rib function and result in rib dysfunction and tenderness in the muscles of respiration.

49. **D Diabetics are acutely sensitive to early signs of ischemia**. Silent ischemia are episodes that can be detected by EKG but occurs without the patient ever perceiving ischemic symptoms. This type of ischemia is very common in diabetics.

50. **A Thoracic lymph pump to increase lymphatic return**. The above patient has pulmonary vascular congestion. Increasing lymphatic return will help decrease the pulmonary congestion. Treating tenderpoints from a viscero-somatic reflex is futile because the pain typically returns within one hour. Redoming the diaphragm will improve respiratory dysfunction, but the CHF is not due to respiratory compromise, it is due to the MI. Correcting thoracic dysfunction with HVLA will restore symmetry but will not have great affects on this patient's CHF. Rib raising will normalize *sympathetic* outflow.

Case K

51. **D Order a urology consult**. General supportive measures include hydration and administration of an analgesic. The KUB demonstrated a 6mm radio-opaque mass. A 6mm stone has approximately a 20-50% chance of being passed, however the IVP demonstrates severe hydronephrosis which may cause a compromise in renal function. Therefore, discharging this patient home would be ill-advised. Since the KUB and IVP confirm the diagnosis of a 6mm stone with hydronephrosis there is no need to do a CT of the pelvis.

52. **A Right psoas tenderpoint**. Due to close proximity of the ureter to the psoas muscle. Renal stones are likely to cause irritation of the psoas. Other dysfunctions listed are possible but are less likely.

53. **A Lumbar somatic dysfunction**. The psoas muscle originates from the transverse processes of the lumbar spine. Therefore, psoas dysfunction is most associated with lumbar dysfunction. Other dysfunctions listed are possible but are less likely.

54. **C Calcium oxalate**. Approximately 80% of all renal stones are calcium oxalate, 5% are uric acid and 1% are cystine, the remainder are magnesium ammonium phosphate or calcium phosphate. Also, uric acid and cystine stones are not easily visualized on a KUB.

Case L

55. **E Nerve conduction and electromyographic studies**. Tinel's, Phalen's and Prayer tests are all used to aid in the diagnosis of carpal tunnel syndrome. However the sensitivity and specificity for these tests vary and therefore not considered diagnostic. Finkelstein's test is positive for tenosynovitis of the abductor pollicis longus and extensor pollicis brevis. Carpal tunnel syndrome is a neuropathic problem and will not show up on a bone scan.

56. **E** **Correction of the cervical somatic dysfunction**. It is best to treat the axial skeleton before treating the upper extremities.

57. **C** **decreased muscle strength in opposition of the thumb**. Compression of the median nerve from carpal tunnel syndrome will result in muscle weakness (abductor pollicis brevis, opponens pollicis, and flexor pollicis) and decreased sensation to the first 3 ½ digits. Sensation to the little finger, and abduction and adduction of the fingers is supplied by the ulnar nerve. Sensation to the dorsum of the hand is supplied by the radial and ulnar nerve. Adson's test will be positive in thoracic outlet syndrome.

58. **C** **T5-T7**. Sympathetic control of the upper extremity is supplied from T5-T7. Although the upper extremity receives innervation from cervical spine, the sympathetic chain ganglia are located only in the thoracolumbar region.

Case M

59. **E** **Muscle relaxants**. Muscle relaxants are not considered first line treatment in patients with temporomandibular dysfunction. Although it is often associated with hypertonic muscles of mastication, muscle relaxants at a therapeutic dose is likely to interfere with the patient's daily activities. [30] Other treatments including heat, OMT, craniosacral therapy and NSAIDS have all been beneficial in treating temporomandibular disorder.

60. **C** **The patient should exercise her jaw by eating chewy foods, like gum or taffy**. The above patient experiences pain and popping while eating. Chewy foods, such as gum or taffy, may worsen the condition. Stretching the muscles of mastication, wearing a bite plate or alternately using heat and ice have all been shown to be beneficial in treating temporomandibular disorder.

61. **D** **CN VIII**. Dysfunction of the vestibulocochlear nerve is most often associated with tinnitus.

62. **C** **TMJ symptoms are present in less than 1% of the population**. TMJ symptoms including popping or clicking is present in approximately 33% of the population. However, only 3-7% seek medical treatment. [30]

Case N

63. **B** **Posterior radial head**. A posterior radial head may present as a sharp pain at the wrist or elbow and may result from a fall on an outstretched arm. On examination, a posterior radial head will be restricted in supination.

64. **D** **HVLA to the wrist to improve range of motion**. Although the X-rays of the wrist are normal, the patient may still have a small nondisplaced scaphoid fracture. The scaphoid bone is the most common bone fractured in the wrist and often presents with pain in the anatomic snuffbox. X-rays may be normal for a week or longer. [29 p.467] HVLA in this case would be contraindicated. Muscle energy, counterstrain, and myofascial release may all be done in this case without worsening the patients symptoms.

65. **B** **Repeat the wrist x-ray, even though the first set was normal. Then immobilize the wrist for three months**. Since x-rays may be normal for a week or longer, it is best to repeat the x-rays and immobilize the wrist with a cast for three months or longer. Due to the lack of a rich blood supply the healing of a fractured scaphoid is characteristically slow. Immobilizing the wrist for two weeks will not allow the fracture to fully heal. Putting the child on a pain medication is ill-advised especially with the likelihood of a fracture. Wrist sprains typically improve with a weeks time. If the swelling and pain are increased, the diagnosis of a fracture should be considered.

Cited References

1. American Osteopathic Association: Foundations for Osteopathic Medicine. Baltimore, Williams and Wilkins, 1997.

2. DiGiovanna, E., Schiowitz, S.: An Osteopathic Approach to Diagnosis and Treatment. Philadelphia, J.B. Lippencott Co., 1991.

3. Moore, K.L., Clinically Oriented Anatomy: Third Edition. Baltimore, Williams and Wilkins, 1992.

4. Brashear, Jr, H.R., Raney, Sr, R.B.,: Handbook of Orthopaedic Surgery. Tenth Edition. St. Louis, The C.V. Mosby Co., 1986.

5. Magee, D.J.: Orthopedic Physical Assessment. Second Edition. Philadelphia, W.B. Saunders Co., 1992.

6. Hoppenfeld, S.: Physical Examination of the Spine and Extremities. Norwalk, Conn., Appleton-Century-Crofts, 1976

7. Borenstein, D.G., Wiesel, S.W., Boden, S.D.: Low Back Pain. Second Edition. Philadelphia, W.B. Saunders Co., 1995

8. Berkow, R.: Merck Manual. Sixteenth Edition. Rahway, Merck Research Laboratories, 1992

9. Buckwalter, J.A., Weinstein, S.L.: Turek's Orthopaedics: Principles and their Applications. Fifth Edition. Philadelphia: J.B. Lippincott Co.,

10. Rubin, A., Stallis, R.: Evaluation and Diagnosis of Ankle Injuries. American Family Physician. 1996;54(5):1609-1618

11. Magoun, H.I.: Osteopathy in the Cranial Field. Kirksville, The Journal Printing Co., 1976

12. Pratt-Harrington, D., D.O., ...Except for OMT! Copyright 1996.

13. Fix, J.D.: Neuroanatomy. Second Edition. Baltimore, Williams and Wilkins, 1995

14. Greenman, P.E.: Principles of Manual Medicine. Second Edition. Baltimore, Williams and Wilkins, 1996

15. Patterson, M.M.: A model mechanism for spinal segmental facilitation. JAOA. 1976;76:62/121-72/131.

16. Berne, R., Levy, M: Physiology. Third edition. St. Louis, Mosby, 1993

17. Guyton, A.: Textbook of Medical Physiology. Eight Edition. Philadelphia, W.B. Saunders 1991

18. Adams, R., Victor, M.: Principles of Neurology. Fifth Edition. New York, McGraw Hill, 1993

19. Owens, C.: An Endocrine Interpretation of Chapman's Reflexes, 1937. Reprinted by the Academy of Applied Osteopathy, May 1963.

20. Travell, J.G.: Simons, D.G., Myofascial Pain and Dysfunction. Vol I. Baltimore, Williams and Wilkins, 1983.

21. Travell, J.G.: Simons, D.G., Myofascial Pain and Dysfunction. Vol II. Baltimore, Williams and Wilkins, 1983.

22. Simons, D.G.: Muscle Pain Syndromes. J. of Manual Medicine, 1991;6:3-23

23. Chaitow, L.: Soft Tissue Manipulation. Ellington, Great Britian, Thorston Publishing, 1987

24. Olsom, W.H., et al.: Handbook of Symptom-Oriented Neurology. Second edition. St. louis, Mosby-Year Book, Inc., 1994

25. DiGiovanna, E., Schiowitz, S.: An Osteopathic Approach to Diagnosis and Treatment. Second Edition. Philadelphia, J.B. Lippencott Co., 1997

26. Yates, H.A., Glover, J: Counterstrain: A Handbook of Osteopathic Technique. Tulsa, Y Knot Publishers, 1995

27. Chung, K.W.: Gross Anatomy. Third Edition. Baltimore, Williams and Wilkins, 1995

28. Kuchera, W.A., Kuchera, M.L.: Osteopathic Principles in Practice. Second Edition. Kirksville, 1991

29. Salter, R.B: Textbook of disorders and injuries of the musculoskeletal system. Baltimore, Williams and Wilkins

30. Okeson, J.P., et.al: Temporomandibular disorders in the medical practice. Journal of Family Practice 1996:13 (1) 347-356

Index

N

P

Q

R